Enter the Ageing Dragon...

中国龙进入高龄化社会…

Musings on the nascent senior living industry in China

中 国 养 老 产 业 初 成 长 的 冥 想

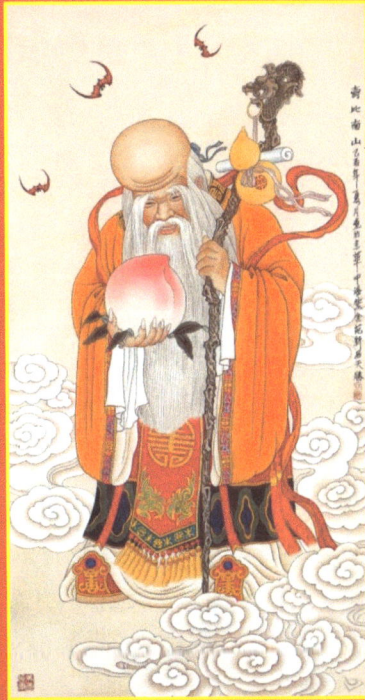

Bromme Hampton Cole

柯 博 明

Enter the Ageing Dragon...

中国龙进入高龄化社会...

Musings on the nascent senior living industry in China

中 国 养 老 产 业 初 成 长 的 冥 想

by

Bromme Hampton Cole

柯 博 明

Published in the USA by: Patient Lao Wai Publications in cooperation with

China Senior Living, ltd

and

Hampton Hoerter Healthcare

ISBN-10: 098568710X
ISBN-13: 978-0-9856871-0-6
Library of Congress: 2013939895
CreateSpace Independent Publishing Platform North Charleston, South Carolina

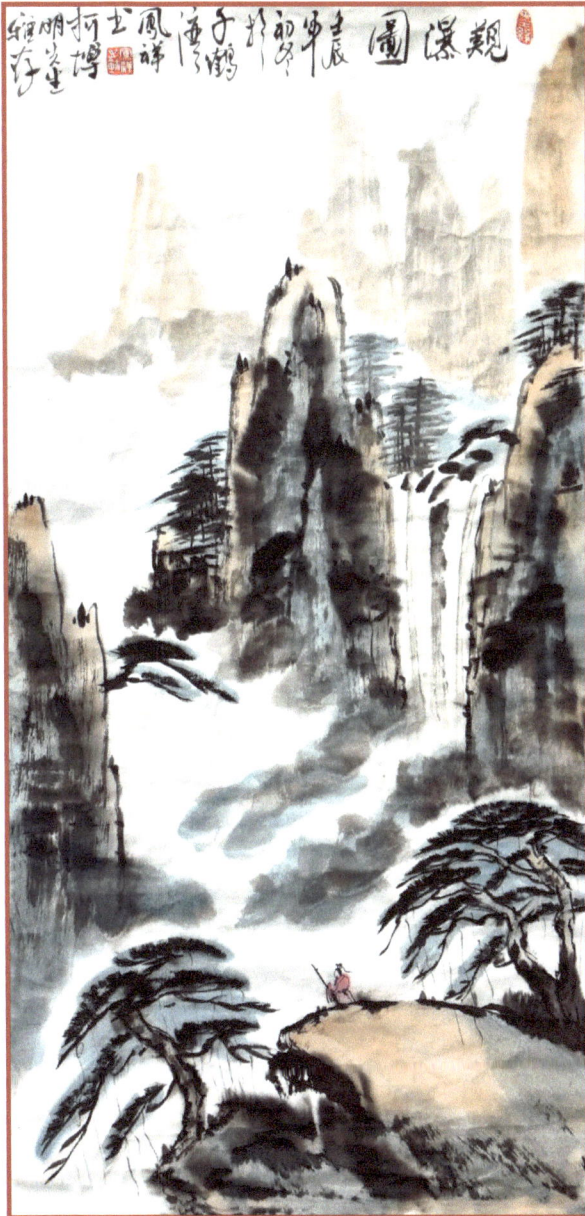

Jiangsu Painting[2]

2 This illustration is by Mr. Li, a businessman, altruistic senior living developer, accomplished artist and good friend who painted it for me on my first trip to Yancheng, Jiangsu province.

This book is dedicated to my three children,
the best kids in the world:

Mackenzie Kathryn

Behold, my first child! A blossoming young lady of peerless poise, incomparable beauty and uncommon intelligence!

Bromme Hampton II

Ah, my son! I am the luckiest father! You are the most talented and handsome young gentleman I have ever met the world isn't ready for you.

Waverly Hayes

And now I have a princess! Mesmerizing beauty, charming wits and supreme confidence all in one delicious package!

I have missed you all terribly during my long sojourns. Hopefully this book, in some small way, compensates for my frequent absences.

* A special remembrance to my young Bao-Mu health care worker, Jiang, wherever you are, Godspeed*

"It is the child that sees the primordial secret of Nature and it is the child within ourselves to which we return. The child within us is simple and daring enough to live the secret." Lao zi

Dear Reader:

While it can be shallow and highly superficial at times, there is also a good deal in popular culture that is enduring and precious. We live in an age of ephemeral entertainment and in our constant quest to be continually amused we risk developing relationships, intimate as well as formal, whose meanings are measured by the extent to which they distract and their commercial value as opposed to emotional content and integrity. Yet, I find solace in that the insipid and transitory nature of present day recreation is offset by a fair amount of profound artistic stimulation, however modern though it may be. Among my personal favorites are contemporary classic literature and their film adaptations; here is where this story begins.

This book is a collection of essays previously published at my website www. ChinaSeniorLiving.com and knitted together with original short stories about my visits to and work in various Chinese cities. Since the original publication of the essays, I have made certain editorial changes but if you read them then you will recognize them in this book. They are artful stories about the early stages of the geriatric care industry in China. I narrate them in the context of a classic movie that has something, directly or indirectly, to do with the country along with an excess of meandering metaphor and ambling allegory all of which I believe delightfully illustrate my adventure here in China. (Ah! But what, I have often wondered, is life without abundant comparative meaning?) However quirky and sinuous the story lines, they are based in reality and founded on fact; thankfully they are not dull as I have done my best to treat this otherwise tedious and sometimes gloomy subject with some wit. Though I will admit, using memorable film to tell stories about China has its limitations. The short interludes which separate the essays, or intermissions as I call them, are intended to be nothing more than refreshing pauses, adding environment, atmosphere and context to the larger series of stories about senior living in China. And, uncomfortable as the subject of ageing and its ultimate destination may be for some, the ominous future of a geriatric planet (much less an ageing China) has implications few, including myself, have fully thought through and for which we all are truly unprepared.

In sum, these essays contain a good deal of experience and observation, both raw and refined.

I have written this book for two reasons; first, I hope it will serve as somewhat of a primer to those interested in entering this business and therefore advance the woefully inadequate standards of Geriatrics in China even when evaluated within the context of rapidly improving Chinese health care; and second, as I witnessed the early days of this industry, I felt a strong need to catalogue and chronicle its development. Having a front row seat for such a transformational event in China's history and at times being a participant, has been and continues to be fascinating. In addition, few of the people in the stories which follow are actual living persons; instead, to accommodate my story lines, I have frequently combined personalities, changed names, compressed timelines and merged experiences. But, generally, the stories are in chronological order and are narratives of real situations; the only exception being a conclusion here or there or an expedition into the future.

And for those not so entrepreneurially inclined to join the fun here in China, approach this book as an adventure story, after all it is all about exploration. I am neither a geriatrician nor a gerontologist but a professional in the health care business...in China, and as of today, an amateur novelist. Doing business in the world that is China is certainly frustrating and full of risk, but the human stories are endearing and the potential financial rewards are great. I wish all who enter the ageing dragon, good luck and above all...the most eminent of all virtues...patience; it will serve you well in China.

Bromme Hampton Cole

Shanghai, March 2013

亲爱的读者：

虽然流行文化有时表现肤浅粗俗，其中也不乏持久且弥足珍贵的片段。我们生活在一个快娱乐的时代。在一心多用追求不间断愉悦的同时，我们有可能在不经意间沉迷于以商业和娱乐价值为导向的人际关系，渐而匮乏真切的情感和高尚的品格。值得慰籍的是在当今乏味而瞬变的娱乐生活的本质中，依然能找到尽管摩登但仍然耐人寻味的文艺气息。我个人钟爱的是当代文学经典和其改编的电影，故事就是从这里开始的。

这本书是由来自我的网站www.ChinaSeniorLiving.com中一组随笔组成，其间穿插了还未出版的关于我在中国多个不同城市的小故事。尽管我进一步编辑了以往的随笔，但老读者还是会在书中看到熟悉的片段。这是些艺术化的关于中国养老产业初期发展的故事。我选择以相关度不一的经典电影为线索，并以婉约的比喻和轻缓的寓言讲述这些故事。（啊！我时常自语，若没有比较，如何能说明生命之意义？）虽然故事中不乏古怪晦涩的地方，但它们的确源于现实，基于事实。作为作者，我尽力用智慧将原本可能有些枯燥或阴沉的主题变得有趣些。老龄化和人生终极这样的话题也许会令人不安。面对这个预兆老去的星球（不仅是中国）很少有人，包括我自己在内，能够真正完全想明白。所以，我们都还没有完全准备好。在这里，随笔能分享的是积累多时的行业经验和观察，以原生或精炼的形式呈现给大家。

我写这本书有两个初衷。首先，希望它能为有兴趣进入该业务领域的人打个基础，借以促进亟需的中国医疗产业背景下养老标准的完善。其次，我觉得针对处于开拓阶段的养老行业有必要捕捉和分享其发展态势。我有幸在这样的时机近观重要事件的发生，并时常参与其中，着实引人入胜。这些故事是以时间为序，以日志的方式阅读即可。

即使您并无创业打算也同样能享受乐趣。这本书有的是冒险故事，毕竟在新行业探索也是种探险。我本人既不是老年医学专家，也不是老年病学权威，我只是养老产业中的一个专注的商务人士......也可以说是位现在扎根于中国的业余小说家。在这里拓展业务并不容易，不乏风险和焦虑。但这些人文故事令人着迷，潜在的经济回报也同样具有吸引力。我忠心祝愿踏上中国龙老龄化之旅的人们好运！

柯博明

上海，2013年3月

注：书的封面是中国神话中的长寿之神寿星。他的站姿平稳，正在愉悦无忧地思考未来。他的右手轻握着一个桃子，是中国文化中代表长寿的仙果。左手他拄着的龙头拐杖，上有仙人的灵物葫芦。寿星身边蝙蝠飞舞，它们象征着好运和福气。但是没人告诉我为什么他有着如此硕大而光亮的额头。我猜测这是长者智慧的象征吧。在众多长生灵物的围绕下，寿星当之无愧是中国养老产业完美的缪斯。

当我初到中国工作的时候，希望能找到业务的方向和意义。偶然发现寿星，这位温和可爱的老者继而成为了我这些年来创意和启发的源泉。事实上，我的第一场演讲就是基于想象中的寿星与福禄两星的对话。如果著名诗人罗伯特•弗罗斯特写一首关于老爷爷的诗，我想寿星会是他笔下极具生命力的角色。

And now for a healthy dose of decorum...

Special thanks to the following friends without whose kindness this book would likely not have happened:

Mom and Dad for their steadfast support and belief in me, Miranda Liao for her excellent Mandarin titles and unwavering support, Elaine Young for the original inspiration to delve into this crazy industry in China...I will never forget your first question to me "Why don't you go to China with all your senior living experience?...", Andrew Oksner for his continued support, humor and supernatural ability to debate a subject objectively and compassionately, Mark "The Godfather" Spitalnik for his ideas and insight, Narinder Dusanj for her blithe spirit, Chairman Yu Ya Ping for being a believer and my first client in China as well as being the inspiration for a certain character in this book, Bin Xiang for his friendship, Susie Bates for her friendship and insight into the Chinese that only 25 years of living here can bring, Tom Hill for his ideas and openness, Jim Biggs for his approachability and friendship, Tania Branigan for being a good egg, Ann Broderick for her friendship, David Collins for his objectivity and editorial acumen, Margaret Connolly for her friendship, support, assistance and constant belief that I was going to make it, Li Ayi and Auntie Joyce for their great food, Michael and Natalie Darragh for being team players, Lilly Donohue for her friendship, Junsong Gao at Yue Cheng for his friendship, Guo Ping for his demographic insights and assistance with my 2012 visa, Lisa Jiang for her friendship and thoughts on food, Josh Johnson for trying really hard, Charles Lam for his patience and interest, Monique Larkin, Adam Lazar, Janet Pierce for her friendship and editorial acumen, Daniel Leaf for being a good dude, Cong Lin for his humor, Christy Yao at Le Amour for being intrepid, Bruce Liu for his help in Taiwan, Ning Lu, Charles Lucas, Trip Dorkey, Don Twiss for his gift of a book on Chongqing and the "Hump", Joseph Christian for a pretty damn good voice and thoughtful commentary, Linda van Ras for her excellent proof reading skills, Danny Ning, Heather Thompson for her friendship, editorial acumen and prodding, Vicky Cheng for always trying so hard and giving me a greatest Mandarin name I could have hoped for, Gomin Kim for being a good analytical modeler, Il Han Kim for being a good writer and a bud, Ies Paalvast, Brad Perkins for all his introductions and knowledge base, Jason Cronk for his insights and editorial acumen, Yvonne Li, Kevin "Mr. T" Ryan for being the best Tosser only another Mr. T could appreciate, Benjamin Shobert for being the only other serious essayist in this industry, Haishan Yang, Ian Montgomery, Serge Kasarda my best friend, Jesse Williamson for his early help, Chris Gardener for sticking with me, Tony Zhao, Janice Chia for loving this industry as much as she loves the beach, the snowy-white haired old lady at PH45 in Chongqing (I didn't mean to scare you!), Romilly Sinclair for asking me to be the first Chairman of RLW China, Ting Ting Wang, Sam Crispin, Susheela Rivers for, well, being Susheela, Beatrice Hsi for some constructive criticism, Rose Noel Pritchard for including me in early MIPIM and MIPIM Asia productions, Christine Lam, Jason Wulterkens for his support, Driver Chen for his punctuality despite the Beijing traffic, Johnathan Sze for his friendship, support and help with business in China, Chris Hu, Mr. Zhang, Min Cole for something but I can't remember what, Michael Coler for his ideas, which, for never having set foot in China are quite good, Richard Price for his early guidance, Coco Chen from Wenzhou for her trust, John Levert for his friendship and guidance in those early days in Hong Kong, the bartenders at Posto Publico on Elgin Street - HK, Karsten Ankjær Jensen, Denmark's Ambassador to China, for his impartiality, the members of the China Senior Living group on Linkedin, Xin Lu for her good work on the HiT contract, Crystine Zhang for the inspiration of her life struggles, Ursula for her care of my three children, Marion La Pierre for appreciating my photographs, Peter Chan at TEC HK, Ray Ashton for having ridiculously archaic views on China, the good men at 69th and Park as well as my Brothers on 23rd and 6th in NYC, the HSNY - Oranje Boven; the Dutch diaspora continues!, my Mandarin teacher Tim Xu, Ann Marie Mourad for visiting China, Shou Xing for being the perfect muse, Richard Hoffman, my 9th grade

English teacher for his favorable comments on my writing way back then, Tricia Cole for so much and random others whose spontaneous kindness inspired me to continue when the going got tough: Whew... thank you all!

Extra thanks to:

Linkedin, UBM - Care Show China, IMAPAC – Retirement Living World, Shama - Peel Street HK, the employees at The Business Centre 3 Pacific Place – HK, the Ding-Ding in HK for transporting me back and forth to the office very inexpensively and ever so romantically.

Extra *special* thanks to:

The 1.45 billion Chinese people who welcomed me to their country and made me feel at home.

Tongue-in-cheek thanks to:

The Chinese government of the late 1970's who legislated the One-Child Policy and, with the stroke of a pen, set in motion a staggering artificial demographic construct, the full consequences of which will be experienced for another 60 years during which China will radically change.

...and Fei chang xie-xie to:

My proof readers: Dad, Mom, Jack Cumming, Heather Thompson

TABLE OF CONTENTS

Table of Figures[2]

---

2 The figures above are photographs, the vast majority of which I took with my Blackberry. There are instances where I have opted for a better photo found on the internet, usually Wikipedia or another source. In the cases where the photo is not original, I note such with the photographer's name, the internet address or when a Wikipedia photo is used, noted as (Wkpd).

Preface by Mark Spitalnik

In 2006, after having lived in China for eight years, it became clear to me that the Chinese tradition of filial piety could not withstand unchanged the demographic and economic trends that were occurring in Chinese society. The one-child policy, in effect in China since 1979, had created a demographic landscape whereby there were less and less young people to care for a growing elderly population while at the same time increasing wealth had resulted in more and more families seeking to "contract out" their duty of filial piety by having third parties provide care to seniors who needed help with activities of daily living. This resulted in a situation where large numbers of Chinese seniors who needed such help and whose families could no longer care for them at home were being cared for in hospital geriatric wards despite the fact that such wards were not designed to provide long term care to those who needed it.

Having been involved with various aspects of the health care business in the United States since 1989 and in China since 2002, I had become familiar with the "culture change" movement - a nontraditional approach to long term care that seeks to transform traditional long term care models similar to those being applied in the geriatric wards of Chinese hospitals into places that genuinely reflect the safety, comfort and pleasures of "home" – and became convinced that many Chinese families would seek to take advantage of a residential aged care solution modeled on "culture change" concepts that envisioned a culture of aging that is life-affirming, satisfying, humane and meaningful in whatever setting elders live. As a result, in 2009, I formed China Senior Care, Inc., with the goal of developing a five-star state of the art residential aged care facility in China. The central tenets of the culture change movement have been built into China Senior Care, Inc.'s mission, vision, and core values.

I met Bromme H. Cole two years after I formed China Senior Care, Inc., while speaking on residential aged care at a conference in Beijing. Since that time,

Bromme has become an important part of the senior care industry in China and a chronicler of its development. Bromme's observations in *Enter the Ageing Dragon*... provide both entertaining and compelling insights into the origins of the nascent Chinese senior living industry that both he and I have been involved. It is my belief that this industry will grow in fits and starts over the next five years, ultimately resulting in a unique Chinese product that will integrate the best of Western senior living concepts with traditional Chinese notions of filial piety; all of which have been modified to meet the needs of a rapidly changing and developing China. *Enter the Ageing Dragon*... provides the reader with a bird's eye view of the journey that those working within the Chinese senior living industry have begun. Its view is from one who has immersed himself in the various challenges entrepreneurs and senior living professionals face as they seek to provide needed homes and services for the ageing. I believe reading *Enter the Ageing Dragon*... will prove of value to those interested in doing business in China as well as and to those who want to better understand the phenomenon of a population ageing and its impact on China.

Mark Spitalnik
President & CEO
China Senior Care, Inc.
www.csc-del.com

Founding Director and President
China Branch, International Association of Homes and Services for the Ageing
www.iahsa-china.org

Li Ma

Li Ma, an 85 year old woman born in Henan province, is beginning to feel her age as she limps across Lu Ban Lu in Shanghai. She steps up onto the sidewalk with her right leg and uses her cane for leverage to boost her bad left leg. She shifts her hips and pivots on her cane, the momentum is sufficient to swing that limp leg up and onto the sidewalk; just in time as a phalanx of motorcycles roar past her. She smiles as she sees me approach and greets me with a soft "Ni hao". In the past year her back has begun to ache and her once sharp brown eyes are now full of smoky cataracts. She is known in the Luwan neighborhood where she lives, as Ma Ayi or Auntie Ma. Auntie Ma was born into a severe famine in Henan province which took her father's life. By the time she was 13, yet another famine, worsened by Japanese war, punished Henan. This time she lost the rest of her family and found herself alone. Soon afterwards, she was hired as a messenger for the Communist Party and eked out a meager living for herself. Fifteen years later she was 31, married and a mother when misfortune struck harshly once again. The Great Chinese famine hit and her husband was one of 30 million who died. 10 years later, during the Cultural Revolution, a middle aged Auntie Ma was involuntarily relocated with her daughter to Shanghai where she was hit by a speeding military truck; the impact broke her leg. The doctor at the hospital set her femur incorrectly and she has limped ever since. For her dedication to the Communist Party she receives a small pension, some health care and a free room in a boarding house which she shares with four other old women. Her daughter is gone; working in a restaurant in far off Hainan.

Li Ma turned and looked at me askew; a foreigner asking all sorts of prying questions about her life. "None of this is his affair", she must think. But Ma Ayi is honest and discloses a life, half full of starvation, war and death. The other half of her life has escaped her, while she was raising her daughter alone China ran away and became a big modern country in which she, and millions just like her, are merely spectators. Yet in our discussions, Ma Ayi never protested her circumstances, voiced no grievances against the life she was given, has no complaints whatsoever. She is content and accepts her position in life as if it were the natural order; she is a simple woman exemplifying ineffable Taoist ideals.

When I met her for the last time, she was on her way to the community health clinic to get her daily dose of heart medicine. It's free, but she must walk 10 blocks and cross two large city highways to receive it. To be sure, a long and arduous trek for an 85 year old woman; but then again, nothing in Auntie Ma's hard life has been a stroll.

Enter the Ageing Dragon.....
中国龙进入高龄化社会...

"Don't think....feeeel. It's like a finger, pointing away to the moon. Don't concentrate on the finger or you will miss all that heavenly glory",
Bruce Lee in **Enter the Dragon**

On the cover of this book there is a picture of Shou Xing, the Chinese deity of longevity. He stands, well-balanced, amused and in worry-free, patient thought about the future. He gently holds in his right hand a large peach, the Chinese symbol for good health and immortality. In his left hand a reassuring staff for those wobbly moments, topped with a dragon head and on which hangs a pumpkin gourd full of life's sweet nectar. Fluttering about him are bats, the presence of which is auspicious in Chinese culture. But no one has ever been able to explain to me his exceedingly large, shiny pate: I can only guess it is emblematic of vibrant mental capacity; yet another important quality for robust old age. Armed with these accoutrements of long life, I find Shou the perfect muse for the senior living industry in China.

When I first began my work in China, I searched for an anchor on which to fix my meditations for the business. I found Shou quite by accident; he is a lovable, gentle old man and my source for numerous inspirations over the years. In fact, the first major speech I gave about senior living in China was via an imagined conversation between him and his fellow deities, Fu Xing and Lu Xing. Shou is the sort of endearing character I imagine Robert Frost would have created had he written a poem about a grandfather.

Introduction

同 志 们 好![3] In late 2009 I began to spend a great deal of time in China as I had heard that China was becoming very old very fast. I learned about this nascent industry quite by accident as I was really focused on business in Indochina at the time. But through a serendipitous meeting at a conference in Ho Chi Minh, I learned about China's colossal demographic phenomenon. Immediately, the concept had the ring of authenticity. This notion coupled with what I knew to be the emergence of a Chinese middle class suggested that there might be an enduring opportunity for senior living in China. Prologue

My conversation at the conference was one of those crystalizing events in life, when everything becomes lucid and the future seems to roll out in front of oneself like a red carpet. Up to that precise moment my professional life had been a jigsaw of mismatched, but profitable experiences. With the advent of an elderly housing opportunity in China, everything suddenly fit together perfectly. No more puzzling about the possibility of personal satisfaction with my vocation; senior living in China was where I was headed. I was certain of this as I had both the requisite experience and sufficient cultural exposure: I had been involved in the elderly housing business for quite some time in North America and I previously lived in Taiwan.

Moreover, the global financial crisis had taken a heavy toll on my business in North America and I was looking for another channel. Over the next few weeks I reasoned that the best entrée would be an advisory/consultancy role as real estate development in China

---

3 This Mandarin phrase, Tong Chiu Hao!, is translated as "Greetings, Comrade!"… and was the salutation used frequently by Chairman Mao when he greeted his fellow communist party members. It was very popular during the Cultural Revolution. The proper response is "Shou Zhang Hao!...or Greetings, Great Leader!

by an expat was not really feasible due to a byzantine approvals process along with the nearly impossible prospect of a foreigner buying land from the government. So it began; I had three good reasons to embark on this venture and by early 2010, I was fully committed.

In hindsight, I am not sure how soon it was after I wrote this first essay that I came up with the idea of using China-themed film as a conduit for my China senior living stories, but I seem to recall it was the result of some considerable frustration with trying to understand how senior living was going to work in China. I reasoned that it might be best to learn more about the Chinese...easily said... but I have known many who lived here their entire lives and still find the people and their culture a mystery. Nevertheless, I wasn't going to be deterred, so I started to read every piece of literature on the subject, studied Confucianism, and watched every movie I could find that had something to do with China. China-themed film captured my imagination in a way that the literature did not. But perhaps most importantly, and something that doesn't reveal itself in the following essays, was my decision to learn Mandarin. Being able to communicate with Chinese on their own terms, using their own idioms and understanding their verbal expressions without the filter of translation is more effective than reading any book or seeing any movie that attempts to reveal the Chinese psyche. Speaking Mandarin means you are no longer a spectator in China and more importantly, earns you the respect of the Chinese, which is only really important if you want to do business here. But first things first...

The film *Enter the Dragon* is perhaps the most successful of all Kung-Fu movies and simultaneously, the peak and the end of Bruce Lee's career. Idiosyncratic and pure genre, it is a David and Goliath movie with lots of chopping, kicking, punching and of course, wuhaaaa-ing. Lee portrays a righteous character bent on avenging his sister's death from a drug overdose at the hands of a local gang. He accepts an offer from the FBI to act as an undercover agent and enters a Kung-Fu tournament held on a fortified island owned by the local drug lord thought responsible for selling the drugs used by his sister. Preposterous feats of supernatural strength aside, the film can in fact teach us something about doing business in China. Consider for a moment Lee's virtue; he exemplifies the archetypal Chinese martyr and embodies classic Confucian philosophy:

> *"Forget a decent haircut, no price is too high to correct the wrong done to my family – Overwhelming odds be damned, if I avenge my sister's death, I will have achieved all that is required of me in this life."*

This self-sacrificial mentality and supreme belief in one's own ability not just to endure but to ultimately surmount any obstacle and vanquish any adversary is distinctly Han. Those doing business in China will encounter this ideal in every Chinese businessman and in every meeting regardless of the industry. In the stories that follow, I attempt to distill this cultural trait and other meaningful ethnic characteristics that I encountered and you will come across as well.

China senior living

In the past 2 years the concept of modern senior living as typically and broadly defined in the West (among three housing categories, independent retired persons, older persons requiring some assistance with chores of daily living and nursing care for the infirm) has become a buzzword in China. This embryonic business has also been perceived as an antidote for the difficulties faced by Western senior living companies that do business in countries with dwindling national pensions, massive government health care funding cuts and cutthroat competition. It seems as though many Western senior living companies think transplanting their operations is simply a matter of translation and licensing. In similar fashion, every Chinese developer has jumped on the senior living opportunity. Their wholesale inexperience notwithstanding, they proceed with making outlandish plans for mega senior living projects. Everyone it seems is rushing headlong into a nascent market that is little understood; the mania is feverish!

A more sober evaluation of the marketplace reveals that there are two competing and parallel realities here: first, there is indeed a demographic opportunity and while it may not be as grand as some say, it is unlike anything the West has seen; second, the economic opportunity, as these things usually go, is much more complex and less clear than the demographic calculus would lead one to believe. As most mania's go, the unbridled and impulsive enthusiasm for senior living will undoubtedly subside as the actuarial intricacies of the business (and many readers will agree that senior living is a business and not real estate) become apparent to local developers and as western geriatric care companies awaken to the difficulties of executing the senior living business in China. Sooner or later everyone pursuing this business in China will reconcile themselves to the following fact:

"Just because a demographic prospect exists doesn't justify or promote an economic opportunity – it needs to be understood, created, marketed and sold on its own merits"[4]

---

4 Bromme H. Cole speech – Retirement Living World China 2011

As a general statement, senior living today in China is being propelled by 3three fundamental forces. Let's examine each:

Demographics: China's well known and highly publicized demographics indisputably show that it is facing a dramatic transition from a young to an aged society in the coming 10 to 20 years. In 2000, there were 88,110,000 persons aged 65 years and older, which represented 7% of the population. Today this figure is closer to 170 million or 14% of the total population; and by 2020 those over 65 will total an astonishing 265 million. There are no official statistics that account for the relative wealth of those in this age cohort, but data and research compiled by my company shows that only about 10.2 million of those aged 65 and older (or their children) have an annual salary of at least RmB1.5 million[5] which gives them the economic means for a private, Western style senior living environment (which says nothing about the interest or motivation or avail themselves of such a living environment). Further and based on a number of conjoint analyses my firm has conducted, this 10.2 million population cohort is also fairly westernized, if not by virtue of their relative wealth, then by travel abroad or via their children who have frequently studied in the West[6].

4-2-1: Because of the peculiar 4–2–1 family structure in China (four grandparents, two children, one grandchild), one can expect that older Chinese adults will increase their use of senior living facilities in the coming years as the burden of one caring for four or six is untenable. With the China's burgeoning economy, the lure of prosperity and the consumerism that follows, it is unrealistic to

---

5 RmB (Reminbi) is the acronym frequently used for the Chinese currency.The conversion rate for a US dollar is approximately 6.2 to 1.

6 I use the term "West" and "Western" to refer to a geography that generally consists of North America, Europe and Australia. I use it also to denote a mindsetor way of thinking that has come to characterize these geographies.

expect that the remaining one child will remain at home to care for the elders. Additionally, the Chinese government has realized that a) it is financially unsustainable to expand in this area indefinitely using public resources and b) they have no real understanding of gerontology as witnessed by the government's stumble with the "Star Light Program" and the "Beloved Care Engineering" launched in the late 1990's and early 2001. Each contained with suboptimal aged care services to say the least. The government's current policy, outlined in both the 12th 5 year plan and the recent Circular 58 and CEPA 67 legislation is to encourage private and foreign investors to participate in the retirement housing business in China. With that said the business opportunities available to foreigners need to be very carefully parsed as nothing is easy in China.

Filial Piety: The Chinese tradition of caregiving for older family members by the younger generation (and specifically the eldest child) is and has always been an inward looking phenomenon; they rely on family members to support all aspects of an elder's care. This is what the Chinese refer to as the value of "filial piety." In fact, China's constitution mentions that "…Children have a duty to support and assist their parents…". While most of the younger persons in China still maintain the attitude that taking care of the older family members is their responsibility, more and more of China's youth are unable and increasingly unwilling to provide all of the traditional family support functions and will therefore require some outside assistance. This is due in part to the 4-2-1 phenomenon mentioned above as well as the impact of China's prosperity and the consequential trend of small nuclear and empty-nest families. It is likely that the traditional concept of filial piety is in transition. It will likely assume a more modern definition that will accommodate a senior living, inter-generational living arrangement homecare or partial care solution.

The mania of senior living in China[7]

The hope of transporting the senior living trend presently emerging in China into an industry is constrained by a single, stark reality;

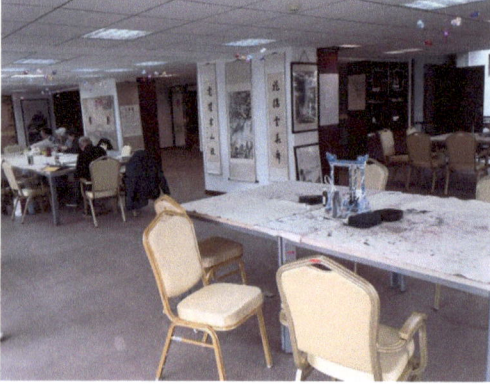

Figure 1 Residents of Cherish Yearn facility practice calligraphy

there is no geriatric health care operator currently in practice in China with the knowledge base that is required to adequately care for a frail, elderly population. Nor is there a cultural norm surrounding this practice. This is not to say that there are no such facilities, indeed there are and at last count, I have found and visited about 35 completed modern facilities. However these facilities are mostly real estate endeavors and/or strictly independent living opportunities with little care services (to wit: Golden Years in Hangzhou). Alternatively, there are facilities that have attempted aged care services but the reality of caring for a frail census far exceeds the ability of the hired staff whose training is simple nursing at best. The point here is something I have spoken at length about in the handful of conferences in Asia on senior living. It is one of the "axioms" of the senior living business in China:

"The tipping point that transforms China senior living from a trend into an industry is the development of "localized" operators who have assimilated and culturally integrated the fundamentals of aged care into an acceptable Chinese

---

7 This passage is largely extracted from an article I wrote for the "German Chamber Ticker", the Business Journal of the German Chamber of Commerce in China,October 2012.

context; simply translating western operating manuals into Mandarin is doomed to fail."[8]

In the senior living business generally, it is critical to distinguish between facilities which offer life style living arrangements and those that are need based. Western geriatric care companies interested in China would be well advised to heed the following: the Chinese demographic that is most attractive and, frankly, the most natural play for Western geriatric professionals is, at present, the mid to high-end of the market that caters to assisted/skilled nursing care facilities (aged care or need based care) and other specialty services such as dementia care. And while there is likely an opportunity at some point for Western companies to get involved with independent senior living (life style) in China, this market has much more local competition. But the more you reduce specialized services, as a Western participant in this industry, the more you diminish your advantage. It is important to note that there are tangential opportunities that should not be overlooked by Westerners in the senior living market here in China. For example, market indicators point to enormous opportunity in the training and education sector as well as the geriatric product supply business; two vastly under represented markets.

> *"The higher acuity level of care which a geriatric services company offers is proportional to its longevity and profitability in China; whereas the extent to which one reduces specialized services, the more you diminish your advantage."*[9]

Yet experience to date has produced ample evidence that this high-end portion of the market is frequently over-estimated. I define the

---

8 Bromme H. Cole, speech at Ageing Asia Alliance, Spring 2011

9 IBID

high-end as senior living `projects with a membership cost of RmB1.5 million (see General's Garden in Beijing) or more, or in the case of a unit sales project, a cost per square meter of RmB20,000 or more. The mid-range is represented by a project with a membership cost of RmB500,000 to

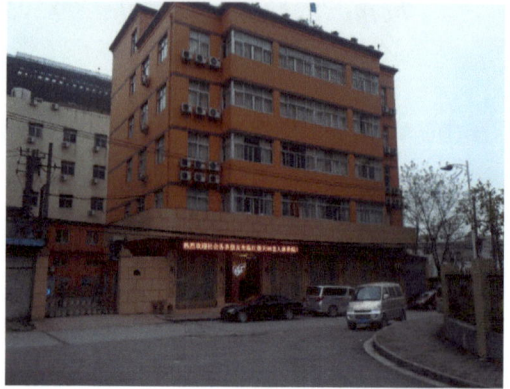

Figure 2 Hong Jin Tian assisted living (high-end) facility in Wenzhou - newly opened

RmB1,000,000 or, again in the case of a unit sales project, a cost per square meter of RmB10,000 to RmB20,000.

For a skilled nursing facility, the high-end is represented by a monthly rental cost of approximately RmB20,000 per month.[10] The low-end of nursing homes, of which there are over 38,000 facilities, offer a very mixed menu of services with little to no consistency in care. In these facilities one can expect to pay anywhere from a few hundred RmB per month to a couple of thousand. There are many examples of free nursing homes although these are often facilities allocated to those disabled in the revolution or other civil conflict. There is really no mid-range skilled nursing facility to speak of, or at least I have been unable to find one (geriatric wards in high-end hospitals which cater to military or political personnel excluded).

Despite all the market chatter and examples which purport to be such, there is no successful high-end life style project in China. In fact, there are a couple examples of very unsuccessful high-end

---

10 The high-end in skilled nursing is being built presently.

attempts (Yanda, for one). What is more, the successful (read: moderately successful but not yet cash flow positive) projects that exist today are solidly at the mid-range of the market: see Cherish Yearn in Shanghai. The reasons for this are just emerging, but I have come to understand it is a function of two fundamental phenomena:

1) No truly 5 star senior living operator exists to complement a high-end facility, so residents are left without meaningful services or a high-end experience; and,

2) Chinese seniors aged 70+ are children of the revolution, civil war, famine…you name it…they have no shortage of traumatic experiences. All of which has made them very thrifty, frugal spenders….even if they are wealthy. Conspicuous consumption and luxury life styles are largely the domain of those born after the death of Mao.

Now an important caveat: specifically excluded from this discussion of success is a needs based product or sub-acute, long term care facility at any end of the market. There is tremendous demand here as every single skilled geriatric nursing facility in China, public or private, has a long waiting list, especially the elite hospitals that cater to high government or military officials. But as much as I see abundant opportunity here, especially for Western operators there are significant obstacles. Yet for those who can persevere and localize operations there is near limitless business potential.

In the long term, I remain very positive with the opportunities for westerners in the China senior living market. The market continues to evolve rapidly and given the mania it is recommended that one remains agnostic especially about the high-end, lifestyle market unless one is willing to invest 3 years in up-front preparation, investigation and just plain learning about what the wealthy Chinese want/need in senior living. Further, the potential over supply and probable slow demand curve concerns me for this market in the near term.

> *"Near-term growth of supply in China senior living assets, particularly the high-end lifestyle product, may significantly outpace demand and if true, the resulting imbalance is likely to persist for the mid-term..."*[11]

Though despite all this rationalization, local developers continue build mega-sized lifestyle projects with plans for on-site, full service hospitals, golf courses and enormous clubhouses; near perfect imitations of what they see when they visit North America or Australia. No amount of well researched local market data will dissuade this phenomenon. It is one of those facts of an emerging capitalist society that compels market participants to expand beyond the capacity of their industry in order to capture or corner the market, or a singular belief in the fallacy of "first mover advantage". This is especially true in China, which has built its success in large part on the rote reproduction of an observed, Western product then manufactured to the point of exhausting the market's ability to absorb. Health care is different, as most of you who are reading this know...it is difficult to imitate. Westerners for their part also continue to insist that they can descend upon the Mainland and establish operations in a year's time using nothing but their existing knowledge base, despite the fact that at least 3 western companies have already shut down operations and left China. All of which underscores just how manic China's senior living mania truly is.

---

11 IBID

Intermission: An American in Chongqing
中场片段: 一个美国人在重庆

When one thinks of China today, the image of some hulking economic and military leviathan stepping up as one of the great powers of the world comes to mind. As China approaches this moment or better yet, as China experiences its renaissance, taking a broader view of the 20th century can provide an initial appreciation for the historically complex relationship between Westerners and the Chinese and a view towards future ones. In doing so it is important to keep in mind that the last 100 years in China

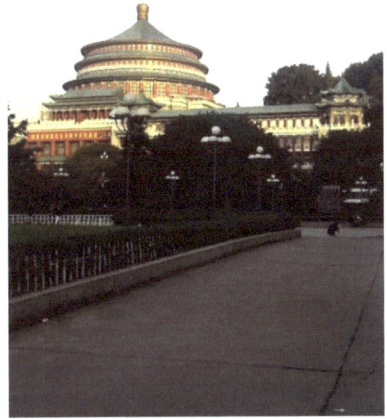

Figure 3 Chongqing Opera house

have been like a misaligned seesaw...pivoting violently from one political and social extreme to another, with momentary episodes of balance which usually end in a nasty war or other alienating chaos. Yet such expansive overviews or comprehensive statements also carry pitfalls; they frequently miss their mark; there is just too much to recapitulate succinctly, too many details whose consequences are far too material to digest in some laconic summary.

So, one good place to begin the focus of this overview, and commence these intermissions, is Chongqing; where I began my work in earnest and a city in which Westerners, and more specifically, Americans and their Chinese counterparts have shared quite a lot. The relationship between them is exemplified by the association which occurred between two men in the early 1940's. The historical experience between this American and his Chinese counterpart was and continues to be a prologue to the future.

Way back then...

For as long as China has been China, Chongqing has been an important city. And today Chongqing is a major urban center in Southwest China and one of the four directly controlled municipalities (directly controlled by the Central government - the other three are Beijing, Shanghai and Tianjin), and the only such municipality in inland China.

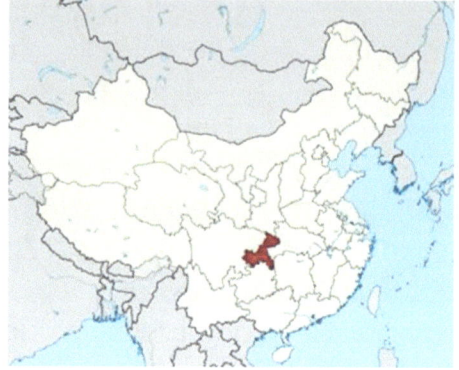

Figure 4 Chongqing (Wkpd)

Chongqing is a large place with a population of about 29 million although the urbanized area is estimated to have a population of about 7 million; it has roughly the land area of North Carolina but with 3 times its population.

In the wake of the Qing dynasty's collapse, the system for governing China was decapitated; central management of the country disintegrated and governance fell to the provinces which in turn gave way to the warlord system that dominated Chinese politics in the 1920's and 1930's. During this period a young, talented soldier named Joseph Stilwell arrived in China with the US Legation, first in Tianjin and later in Beijing. Stilwell was a West Point graduate and a terribly complex man. He was a skilled tactician with a rebellious streak and, however brilliant, his personality lent towards caustic and abrasive behavior. As a General, he eschewed the trappings of high military rank, disliked ceremony and always preferred wearing uniforms without insignia. The quintessential pragmatic general, Stilwell was equally devoted to his mission as he was to his men (albeit harshly); little else mattered.[12]

At the outbreak of World War II, China was effectively under the command of Generalissimo Chiang Kai-Shek, commander of Nationalist Chinese forces and President of the Kuomintang party (KMT). Stilwell, with all his China experience to date, was appointed by Roosevelt as Chief of Staff to General Chiang sent to Chongqing. In addition to US forces in the area, his command was significant and included the Chinese 5th and 6th armies in Southeast China.

General Stilwell participated in a series of military campaigns during his time in China. The Japanese had effectively obstructed supply routes into China along her eastern seaboard and therefore, provisions for the allied military forces had to arrive via Chongqing after being flown over the notorious "hump" from India. This route however was at risk as the Japanese had also invaded Southeast Asia and now were threatening a full, choking blockade of China. The job of securing this supply route and pushing the Japanese out of Burma fell to Stilwell and those under his charge[13] including the Chinese forces. During this time, he and cemented a profound friendship with the Chinese people, training many of the forces personally and fighting side-by-side, though his relationships with his fellow generals, especially Chiang, were often very tense.

---

12 My thoughts on Stilwell come from two sources: 1) Barbara Tuchman's Stilwell and the American experience in China, and 2) Stilwell's personal diaries which can be found at Stanford University's Hoover Institution or http://www.hoover.org/library-and-archives/collections/east-asia/featured-collections/joseph-stilwell.

13 Stilwell was assisted by the famous Chindits (a professional army run by General Wingate), British forces under command of Mountbatten, and the Flying Tigers under General Chenault.

Chiang Kai-Shek came to power as a result of President Sun Yat-sen's death; he was married to Sun's sister-in-law. The Generalissimo was an old school politician and attempted to maintain his grip on power through a system of patronage and playing one warlord off another to ensure his survival. But the one group of people he had absolutely no use for were the Communists, doubtless because they opposed the moneyed class which bankrolled him. Yet for all Chiang's efforts to hold things together after President Sun's death, the KMT soon split with Sun's wife siding with the communists and Chiang's former colleague now adversary, Wang Jingwei, tearing away a portion of the KMT.

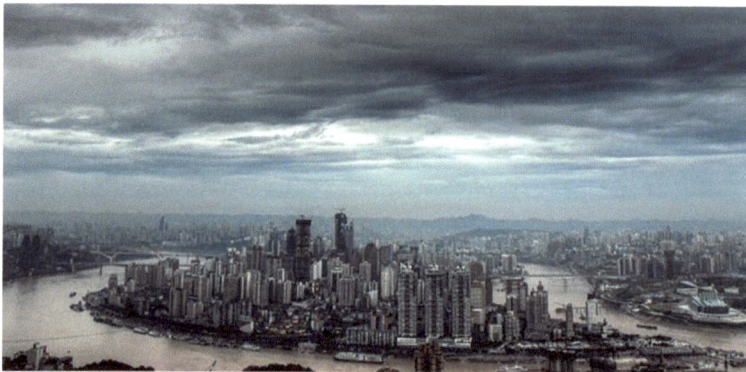

Figure 5 Oblique view of present day downtown Chongqing, looking north (Wkpd)

When it came to China's future, the history shows that both Roosevelt and Stilwell understood that China was destined to become a great power. Roosevelt was convinced of this through the experience of his mother's family (they were missionaries) and Stilwell, through his own knowledge of the industrious ways of the Chinese with whom he fought side by side on the front lines. Roosevelt also wanted to help China's entry onto the world stage. But with Chiang that was difficult. He was his own worst enemy; his method of holding total power prevented him from allowing a successful military figure emerge from among his Chinese generals, his blatant corruption and skimming of American aid (Stilwell's notes reveal an estimated USD$380 million taken by Chiang) as well as a passive-aggressive military strategy that relied largely on allied powers to fight the Japanese while conserving the majority of his troops for an eventual battle against the communists. This sorely irritated those who were trying to help him the most, notably the proactive and mission-oriented Stilwell. Much of Stilwell's energy in southwestern China was allocated to struggles with "Peanut" (the code name for Chiang Kai-Shek) over military strategy. Nevertheless, to his credit Stilwell was able to get enough authority over enough troops to win a major battle against the Japanese in Burma;[14] which victory opened a larger flow of supply to China by over land via a route to become known as the Stilwell Road.

After the defeat of the Japanese in Burma and in an effort to preserve momentum the Americans had won, Roosevelt asked Chiang to make Stilwell the commander over the entire Chinese army. Unfortunately this had the expected result of a loss of face for Chiang who had no other choice but to agree. He acquiesced with one condition: replace Stilwell. Roosevelt complied and installed General Albert Wedemeyer. Stilwell's impressive but turbulent career in China was at an end.

It is apparent that American diplomacy in China during this time was frustrated with the KMT leadership. In fact, one could conclude that the biggest factor which contributed to the loss of China, other than the Japanese invasion which wholly absorbed allied focus and the collective societal realities of China stemming from centuries of dynastic rule, was the KMT government as led by Chiang Kai-Shek. Stilwell himself was so irritated with the Generalissimo that he was certainly ready to consider working with the Communists. He even

---

14 Myitkyina, located on the Irrawaddy River, 1944

hints at times that the Chinese might not be truly communist, but more a people exasperated with the abuse suffered upon them by the Qing. So much so that the "brotherhood" which Mao preached and the stability of the harmonious society it (and he) promised was very appealing. Even the Soviets were never really convinced of Mao's Communist purity, which partially explains why the Chinese and Russians never really developed as enduring allies.

Yet for all the American diplomatic suspicions that proximity to the Chinese communists might prove more productive, i.e., leading to a faster end to the war and a longer term economic relationship as well, it presented a difficult political endeavor back in Washington given the American pre-occupation with the "red-scare". The fear of communism instilled in the West by Bolshevik revolution of 1917 along with the concurrent rise of McCarthyism would have made any such diplomacy next to impossible.

And now…

At #63 Jialing Xin Lu, a winding road which leads from the shores of the Yangtze river up the side of a hill to Eling Park in downtown Chongqing, sits the former residence of General Joseph W. Stilwell; now a museum in honor of his contribution to Chinese liberation. It is a three-storied house with an office, adjutant room, a couple of meeting rooms and a few bedrooms. The houses' simple furniture is arranged as it was during the time that he and his wife lived there, and more than one hundred articles the Stilwell's daily life are on view. In the residence's courtyard, a monument stands in the center on which is engraved an epigraph in both English and Chinese. The words were written by Franklin Delano Roosevelt on May 17, 1944. There is a commanding bust of General Joseph W. Stilwell to one side of the monument, which gives visitors a stark portrait of this iconic man.

It is way too premature to suggest that the teeter-totter of China's economy and political machine has found equilibrium on its societal fulcrum; it certainly hasn't yet. For one, Mao's harmonious society hasn't really offered the concord he promised. It did however produce continued poverty under a very forced unity. But instead of suffering a Soviet like disintegration, the China seesaw swung the other way in the 1980's. Forward thinkers such as Deng Xiao Peng harnessed the potential of China and avoided yet

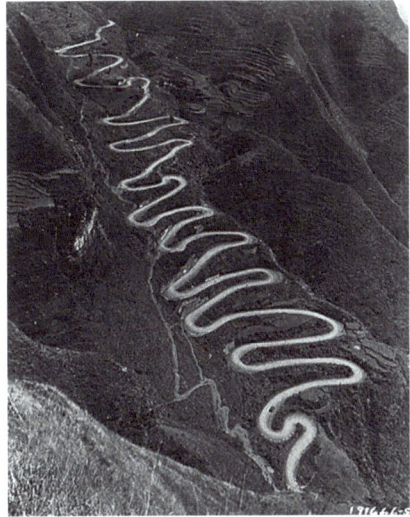

Figure 6 A portion of the Stilwell Road (Wkpd)

another violent era. For another, there remain strong undercurrents of social discontent with the lack of civil rights, limited social programs and, of course that degenerate link which today's China shares with its Dynastic pass: corruption. How intensely the seesaw pivots back in the near future is to be seen.

The painful details of World War II history aside, the story of Stilwell in China reveals all the telltale pitfalls and benefits of Western-Chinese relationships. The pitfalls are obvious: Stilwell was not immune to frustrations stemming from Chiang's corruptions, ambiguous agendas and the all-important, concept of face. Likewise Chiang was no doubt exasperated with Stilwell's impatience; insistence on daily advancement and productivity, his moralizing about the unexplainable costs incurred under Chinese management style and of course, indifference to guanxi. These disparities are universal; they existed then, they are present when I do my business and they will be there for you. Not in any small way, these issues characterize our relationships with the Chinese. How we manage them defines both our successes and our failures. Certainly Stilwell's inability to reach Chiang on his level prematurely ended his career and Chiang's pride and obstinacy contributed to his loss of China.[15]

The benefits however, are embedded in the question which this history affords us: how first to recognize our biases and then overcome these prejudices, or at least relegate them to less than threshold matters, in order to win the deals we attempt to strike.

---

15 Were Stilwell and Chiang here to respond this this conclusion, the American General would no doubt reply in characteristic, steadfast fashion that the preservation of his career was not mission-relevant: he routed the Japanese in Myitkyina and opened up a secure logistics /transport route to China; that is all that mattered. Chiang, on the other hand, would likely point out that he never surrendered to the Communists and laid the foundation for the mightily successful and democratic Taiwan; history has many facets. I find both valid points.

The Joy Longevity Club
喜 寿 会

"I wanted my children to have the best combination: American circumstances and Chinese character. How could I know these two things might not mix well?" Lindo Jong in **_The Joy Luck Club_**

The Practical Challenges of Cultural Translation

同 志 们 好! Throughout Amy Tan's *The Joy Luck Club*, the various female narrators meditate on their inability to translate concepts and sentiments from one culture to another. The incomplete cultural understanding of the mothers and the daughters is a result of their incomplete knowledge of the other's language. Indeed, the barriers that exist *between* the mothers and the daughters are often due to their inability to communicate with one another. Although the daughters know some Mandarin and the mothers speak some English, communication often becomes a matter of translation, of words whose intended meaning compared with their accepted meaning are in fact quite separate, leading to subtle misunderstandings with big consequences.

I could transcribe the above paragraph nearly word for word and have it apply to a western company's experience in bringing their business to China, especially senior living or geriatric health care. This experience for many has been frustrating and this is almost entirely due to each party's inability to understand that the translation being provided for them at the banquet table is imperfect. Each party departs that table with a partial comprehension of the conversation that transpired; yet the perception is that they understood all of what was said. The reality is that both parties understood their translators. Like the mothers and daughters in *The Joy Luck Club*, it is also fair to say that the misunderstanding between an American businessman and his Chinese counterpart is not relegated to the superficial; in fact they approach their meetings assuming they are very different and neither of them realizes that they have more in common than not. Consider for a moment that these two have richly mixed identities rather than identities of warring opposites.

Said another way, the differences between American culture and Chinese culture can be summed up as follows:

Consider China a high-context culture (by context, I mean the whole situation, background, or environment connected to an event, a situation, or an individual) in which the individuals have internalized meaning and information, so that little is explicitly stated in written or spoken messages. In conversation, the listener knows what is meant; because the speaker and listener share the same knowledge and assumptions, the listener can piece together the speaker's meaning. China is a high-context culture.

In contrast, a low-context culture is one in which information and meanings are explicitly stated in the message or communication. Individuals in a low-context culture expect explanations when statements or situations are unclear, as they often are. Information and meaning are not internalized by the individual but are derived from context, e.g., from the situation or an event; America is a low-context culture. At some point because we are all human, low context culture communication meets high context culture communication; this stratum is not a bright line but a seam that is broad and contains meaning and perspective to both cultures.[16]

---

16 This high context/low context discussion comes from Lilia Melani of Brooklyn CUNY.

When American businessmen fear that the American and Chinese cultures cannot mix and therefore doing business in China is perilous, they are contemplating the combination of two extremes of the high/low context dynamic. In reality, each identity is itself mixed: just as the American culture is not wholly about autonomy, liberty and individuality, the Chinese culture is not wholly about passivity, obedience, and self-restraint. Nonetheless, the challenge of finding a way to combine aspects of both into a successful venture is a challenge faced not only by the American businessman in China but also by the Chinese businessman in America. A successful meeting of these two mentalities requires a long term commitment to understand each other, and of course patience.

Membership in The Joy Longevity Club

There are four fundamental principles of working in China which I have found to be essential to beginning to understand the Chinese. This last phrase, "understanding the Chinese" is the catch here and it leads me to the frustrating and slightly contradictory and circular statement that one must understand the Chinese culture before you can understand the Chinese. It is a rich, complex culture with boundless mysteries all of which have been developed over the past 5,000 years. And more recently, Chinese character has been shaped by unimaginable hardship with no fewer than 6 famines, 8 wars. So, understanding the Chinese and their approach to business is really predicated on knowing their history. Nevertheless, I have developed four principles, which I call the "Four philosophies of The Joy Longevity Club". These principles regard situations and people which you will inevitably come in contact with; these principles will help you and, set forth tongue in cheek, are below:

1) **The man with a hundred wives:** He's a clever and oh-so-polite chap. He squeezes Yuan from stones. He's got

a piece of every action imaginable; the taxi driver's fare he hailed to take you to the hotel, the lunch he "paid" for, and if money changes hands within his sight, he has a cut. He is not dishonest; he is the pinnacle of an entrepreneur, the ultimate broker and China is full of them. Do not get angry with him; be his friend, know him…as such is a first step in understanding him and using his considerable network and rich guanxi for your gain.

2) **False-positive affirmation of non-confirmation:** Here's simple axiom for doing business in China, learn it, internalize it and life will be much simpler for you: Yes means maybe, yes can also mean no and yes might indeed mean yes but no invariably means no…..got it? Don't be frustrated, just practice and master this sly bit of linguistic subterfuge and you are half-way there….maybe.

3) **Same-same but different:** This is a disarmingly innocent but crafty little riddle that really only serves a person to advance a particular situation at another's expense. All I can offer you here is the following guidance: "At what point in time are two dissimilar objects identical?" The answer: "When the person who is using this phrase is desperate to convince you of something." But be especially concerned when the attorney you've hired to represent your interests says the same thing to you about a matter of Chinese law. Usually the use of this phrase means that your powers of critical thinking are paying off….the questions you are asking are exasperating him…..keep it up.

4) **General Copycat's spicy chicken with tasty sauce:** This is the main meal that has nourished the Chinese economic miracle. Here is the recipe: In China, the first generation of copied product is a blatant failure while the second is an improvement and works but is

still commercially unacceptable. The third generation however is an inferior product but marketable and the fourth is nearly indistinguishable from its foreign counterparts in nearly every respect except for one: it is much less expensive. This last point, the cost of the product being substantially less, is the point of liminality when the Chinese "gotcha".

Here is an example of a practical application of the above principles. I was recently at a Chinese banquet, the guest of a successful man who owns a large company and was looking to get involved with senior housing; I'm interested in selling him some consulting business. Here is how the conversation went:

Bromme 柯博明[17]: Attempting to demonstrate proficiency with chopsticks, I remark in high context language, "Mr. Chang your interest in senior housing is quite timely and I like your project's location."

Mr. Chang: Displaying supreme ability with chopsticks as he draws his spicy chicken nearer, he says "Xie-Xie. We have diligently been preparing for our opening."

Bromme 柯博明: ….."Opening?" The slippery chicken I had managed to pinch with my chopsticks drops back onto my plate, splattering my shirt with spicy sauce. "I was under the impression you were interested in receiving our proposal for strategic operations assistance?"…I stammer, in full retreat with low context language.

---

17 柯博明 is my name in Mandarin. It is pronounced Ker Boh Ming and, roughly translated, means "clear/bright understanding".

Mr. Chang: Never taking his eyes off his plate, he devours his chicken, gnawing voraciously on the bone. He responds with false-positive affirmation of non-confirmation, "Yes!"

Bromme 柯博明: Batting away the subterfuge, I penetrate, "How can we help you Mr. Chang?"

Mr. Chang: Smiling broadly and gesturing to the waiter that he is finished with his chicken, he says, "We return from our USA trip where we visit two senior facilities. We took a lot of pictures! We would love to read your proposal."

Bromme 柯博明: Mr. Chang's hundred wives are useless against me now! I counter with a masterful Same-Same but Different tactic, "Ah, this is a clever move Mr. Chang and I am sure you learned a great deal. What you learned on your trip will be of great use….." I pause to release the obligatory burp that demonstrates my deep satisfaction with the taste of the chicken…exhaling, I continue,"… especially…. your newly found knowledge of geriatric nutrition and memory care".

Mr. Chang: On his heels and defensive, using False Positive Affirmation of Non-Confirmation, he simply responds, "Yes."

Bromme 柯博明: At this point I must enable Mr. Chang face, I reply in high context language, "Your knowledge of this industry will make you an icon of China senior living! I only hope to offer you support in this voyage, Mr. Chang."

As it turns out, Mr. Chang not only thought he could build a skilled nursing facility using pictures but he had plans to establish a hospital as well….also based on the pictures they took on their recent visit to the US. After an initial attempt at replicating a facility from pictures, Mr. Chang quickly became a client. Fortunately for the geriatric health care consulting business and Western geriatric care companies, the fourth generation of SNF/ALF and liminal profitability for the Chinese is 10 years away.

Mr. Chang's North American counterpart is a man named Cheskel Schoetz,[18] a highly successful senior living developer and owner/operator. I had known of Cheskel and his accomplishments for some time but had never met him during the time my business was based in New York. As life works, I would now meet him in China as he was coming to visit a project for which I had written a large strategic plan and was looking for joint venture partners and investors.

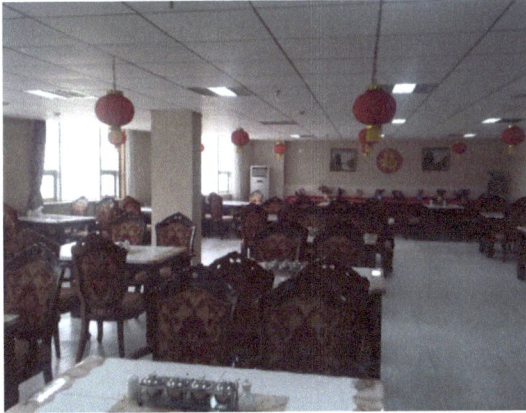

Figure 7 Dining room at Le Amour senior living center in Beijing

Cheskel and his entourage arrived in China and after introductions and the obligatory meal we began the tour of the project the next day. After seeing the land on which the project will be built we also visited other senior living projects in the area. Now, before we began the comparable properties tour and knowing that Cheskel had never been to China before, I tried to prepare him for what he was about to see. But Cheskel being Cheskel, a single-minded and slightly egocentric person, would have none of my advice. I was

---

18 I have changed the name here.

becoming a little apprehensive as my client had hired a number of translators to mingle about the crowd and report back to him on what was being said.

From the moment we arrived at the first property to the instant we left the fourth and final facility, Cheskel was highly critical of everything he witnessed. From landscaping to building design, from interior fit-out to perceived quality of care and services, Cheskel and his minions were almost belittling in their commentary. His conclusion? Everything was wrong. It was not mean-spirited, just condescending and more importantly, ignorant of the situation; like many other Westerners, Cheskel failed to appreciate the embryonic state of Chinese senior living and measured everything he saw in the context of his upscale developments on the East coast of the US. This is understandable, but an improper way to assess and ultimately a terminal error. Cheskel's disdain for what he was witnessing kept him from appreciating the opportunity in front of him. Unfortunately, his comments were passed along to my client by the translators. Subsequent discussions during day were chilled and the dinner that evening was mechanical and awkward.

Cheskel returned to the US and never came back. But even if Cheskel had the humility and presence of mind to understand what he was seeing, I doubt he would have been successful in China anyway. And I say this for reasons I will discuss in later chapters.

Now, a serious word about the future

With all joking aside, explosive economic growth fueled by cheap labor has been the major driving force behind every industrial sector in China; and the health care industry is no exception. The country represents one of the most rapidly growing major health care markets in the world with total health care spending having produced compounded growth of nearly 23% over the past four years making China the fifth largest health care market in the world. And with its current momentum, many expect China to surpass Japan by 2013 to become the second largest health care market in the world. If that isn't enough, China's health care expenditure accounted for a microscopic 4.6% of its GDP in 2009, well below the global average of 10%. By way of further comparison, it's East Asia and Pacific neighbors spend 6.3% of their GDP in health care; so the potential growth is obvious.[19]

China's increasing affluence has brought upon it a frightening rate of urbanization. Accompanying this urbanization are natural lifestyle changes such as western diets, modernized transportation, and intensified work schedules; all of which tend to shift disease patterns from communicable to chronic. These shifts increase demand for recurring health care treatment, especially in older adults whose bodies are less resilient. I believe there is opportunity for Western companies to get involved with senior living in China, but the strategy requires serious market analysis, understanding and preparation prior to any implementation. So, while the economic story is compelling one of the real difficulties in China is execution and, of course, communication or mastering the low context culture vs. high context culture dynamic. For Western geriatric care companies, membership in The Joy Longevity Club is exclusive and takes time.

19 Drawn in near totality from Cowen and Co. Hong Kong research, 2011.

Intermission: A Jigger Full of Guizhou
中场片段: 贵州干杯

The provincial capital of Guizhou is Guiyang, a small third-tier city of about 5 million Chinese. Guizhou was one of Mao's Red Army strongholds; they were endlessly faithful and supported Mao without hesitation through some of his more difficult days. Today, Guizhou struggles to find its share of the Chinese miracle and were it not for the Government's renewed efforts to promote the economies of third-tier cities, Guiyang would not have a new airport, new highway system and a massive "new" downtown developed only a few kilometers from the old city.

The province of Guizhou is pretty; it is a southern province, it is warm and its landscape is dotted with attractive foliage covered, limestone spires or karsts, a geological oddity frequently found in southern China and northern portions of Vietnam[20]. Although some Guizhou organizations do

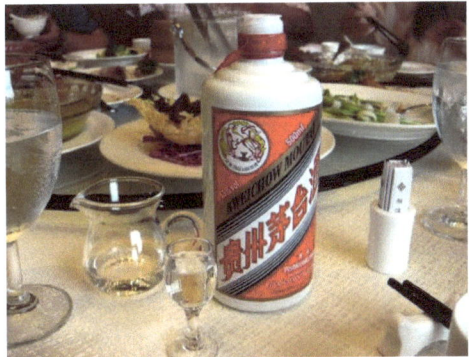

Figure 8 Moutai being consumed at dinner.

attempt to promote the natural beauty of Guizhou in order to attract tourists, many others forego this aspect of the province in deference to another of its products: the notorious yet highly revered Moutai; a clear, 50 proof alcohol made of sorghum. It is powerful…it is an acquired taste…and it is very Chinese. Truth: one will never, baring religious observance, spend much time in China or engage in much business without drinking one's fair share of Moutai; it is a cultural sacrament.

20　To wit: Ha Long Bay near Hanoi.

I was in Guizhou at the invitation of two men, one of whom was the local representative of the Ministry of Railroad's business interests and a Guiyang real estate developer; a combination of personalities that, when found in Guizhou, guarantees that one will consume copious quantities of Moutai at every meal…except breakfast, I hoped.

I arrived in Guiyang on a rainy Tuesday and as the plane wrestled its way through a light storm, searching for the runway in dense fog, I could make out from the window next to my seat many of those karsts formed eons ago. Today, too much regret and environmental insensitivity, these beauties of China's geological past are often merely sources of rock filler for yet another airport runway or superhighway.

We landed with a hard crunch. Twenty minutes later I made my way out of the airport to a warm welcoming ceremony my hosts had arranged. After formalities we were swiftly managed into cars and away to our hotel for a rest and, I feared, to prepare for a lavish banquet with Moutai of course.

My hosts were young men, around 35-40 years old…and they could drink. Round after round after round the Moutai flowed; small 1 ounce jiggers, filled to the brim with what soon begins to taste the way turpentine smells; acrid, noxious and combustible. That evening, I constantly worried about the incessant lighting of cigarettes possibly igniting Moutai fumes. Around midnight, I gave up…I could drink no more. I was teetering on the edge of perception. To applause and compliments for my ability to drink, I staggered back to my room thinking that if Moutai has one saving grace it is that it is fairly pure not unlike vodka; hangovers are mild at worse.

I woke up late and met my clients downstairs for breakfast; my stomach was raw. To my immediate horror, as I sat down for a warm bowl of congee...there was a jigger full of Moutai at the head of my plate.

My hosts smiled and raised their glasses.

Good morning, Guizhou...

Crouching Telemedicine, Hidden Opportunity
"远 程 监 控 医 疗 护 理" 蕴 藏 无 限 商 机

*"No growth without assistance. No action without reaction. No desire without restraint" Mu Bai in **Crouching Tiger, Hidden Dragon***

同 志 们 好! There is no shortage of metaphor in Chinese culture. From language to art, it is a highly philosophical society and one that loves affirming, often in extravagant ways, its traditional values; the Chinese are also quick to turn and embrace the latest technological innovations with a coy wink and a nod. This seemingly mild contradiction between reverence of the past and infatuation with a cutting edge lifestyle is a mystery of sorts. But why not? The Chinese love ambiguity and are not troubled in the least by incongruity.

In Ang Lee's blockbuster Wuxia epic, *Crouching Tiger, Hidden Dragon*,[21] there are many poignant moments in which to drift away in endless contemplation of China's mysteries. Yet one moment stands out in particular: The chief protagonist of the film, Mu Bai, knows that clinging to his personal affection for Shu Lien is contrary to his Wudan way of detachment; yet in Shu's company he finds something that has eluded him in his meditations. In their second key exchange, during the film's midpoint, Mu Bai goes so far as to take Shu Lien's hand and press it to his cheek; yet even here he is held back by the implications of his strident, warrior philosophy. A moment later, in an uncharacteristically romantic moment that underscores Mu Bai's Wuxia code of ethics, he peers into Shu Lien's eyes and says,

---

21 Throughout this book the film descriptions have been drawn, at times heavily, from a number of sources such as Wikipedia, Rotten Tomatoes and others.

"Shu Lien, the things we touch have no permanence....there is nothing we can hold onto in this world. Only by letting go can we truly possess what is real."

Ah.....here we have it all, the Chinese to a T...enigmatic, impenetrable...and perhaps inconsistent but always attractive and enticing.

In a way, and maybe a tad stretched, I find Mu Bai, his words and his actions relevant, almost allegorical to China's health care evolution and in particular its epic, Wuxia-like journey to self-actualize geriatric medicine. Like Mu Bai, who struggles to reconcile his affection for Shu Lien with his Wudan discipline, the story of China's senior health care evolution is cryptic and captivating at the same time; always searching for an elusive goal but restrained by a reluctance to let go of the past only to possess, as Mu Bai lectures, what is real. This pursuit of the abstract for some durable conclusion or permanent truth and the attainment of such, at the price of one's culture, is what I call a "Mu Bai reality".

Today, across China, developers are waking up to the opportunities for senior living and they are not dissimilar to entrepreneurs everywhere; aggressive and acting to fill a demand or enrich themselves by acquiring more and more land. Many of these developers are experienced builders, but most of them do not possess the skill set necessary to offer the elderly tenants the care and service expected....much less initially promised. Further, when few if any industry wide regulations exist to standardize a product, the results can be "consumer unfriendly", meaning seniors are moving into communities without any meaningful care regimes and no near term prospect for such. And since there is no established geriatric care practice, much less regulations for such in China, elderly consumers don't really know what they don't have.

Fortunately, this practice is changing as Western senior care providers begin to investigate the market and as China herself, learns the science and the art of elder care. China's senior health care evolution in this sense is highly transitional and lacks permanence at presence; it is in a sense very embryonic. One might imagine China's senior care industry pupating within a chrysalis comprised of western geriatric competence, modern technologies and traditional Chinese medicine. As it grows, it undergoes a profound metamorphosis; a transformation that requires it to release a portion of its cultural history in order to evolve. The question is: what does it shed and into what does it evolve? When China senior care industry releases and "let's go", as Mu Bai implores Shu Lien, what will it possess and what will it be?

The "Mu Bai reality" of China's senior health care

When I think about the size of the population in China that (today) requires some sort of specialized geriatric attention and likely goes without, I am reminded of the Law of Large Numbers. If I were to envision a perfect world where every senior citizen in China could avail themselves of a senior living opportunity if they needed it, whether it be nursing, independent or assisted living, I would be dreaming of over 350,000 facilities. This is, to say the least, fiscally impractical and likely impossible even for a "China-sized" national budget. So, I wonder, "What is the solution?" Well, the Law of Large Numbers (a theorem dictating that results obtained from a large number of trials should be close to the average of a single trial) tells me that the expected solution for all is not far from the average solution for delivering senior care to 170 million Chinese elderly.

The average solution and the answer, I believe, enabling geriatric care (to non-terminal, ambulant persons) to cover 95% of China's ageing population will be one that utilizes information and communication technology (ICT) to monitor, diagnose, evaluate and maintain patients. ICT is simply a combination of information and communications technologies and is used as a general term for all kinds of technology which enable users to create, access and manipulate information. China is an increasingly interconnected country, the interactions among devices, systems and people are growing geometrically. Businesses need to meet the demands of their employees and customers to allow for greater access to systems and information: ICT enables all of these communications needs to be delivered in a unified, scalable way. This unified platform reduces costs and boosts productivity across a business and beyond. ICT has merged into most every aspect of daily life in China from commerce to leisure and even culture; witness the ubiquity of mobile phones, desktop computers and hand held devices. In most respects, save political, ICT is making China a global society, where people can interact and communicate swiftly and efficiently (albeit there is still an astonishing lack of transparency and censorship remains rampant). There is no mystery here, in an abstract sense, ICT became part of China's technology "Mu Bai reality" in the 1990's when it "let go" of parts of its past.

The health care expression of ICT is Telemedicine. It is a relatively simple concept whereby a doctor can remotely assess the health of a person using devices which measure numerous criteria such as blood pressure, glucose level, temperature, weight and others. These devices already exist, and some manufacturers are producing "all-in-one" portable combinations that sit on top of a table facilitating ease of use. After the device performs its user administered measurements, the data is transferred (wirelessly or via internet connection) to a central assessment unit for interpretation and comparison with personal historical data. If necessary, the doctor can contact the patient via VoIP and if sufficient broadband is available, live video discussion can ensue for greater evaluation. It is estimated that a doctor can "visit" and assess hundreds of patients a day via Telemedicine, dramatically reducing costs by restricting real office visits or home visits to those patients who truly require in-person evaluation. To my mind there are 5 compelling reasons[22] why this technology works:

1) Telemedicine can increase effectiveness and efficiency in geriatric medicine,
2) Currently available technology is sufficient,
3) Remote central assessment units can be located within a hospital or other existing clinic,
4) Technology transforms seniors from patients to consumers,
5) It offers greater quality of life for seniors by maintaining personal independence and the continuity of living at home.

But just because Telemedicine "works" or that ICT is a viable application enabling greater access to health care, why will it work in China? The economic answer is because the majority of elderly Chinese are not rich, will never be rich or live in remote areas and thus are unable to afford a specialized, live-in, dedicated facility or to travel to a doctor on a frequent basis. Not even under some contemplated, distant reality of a Chinese social security or pension system will most of these people have such an arrangement. So, the least expensive, most practical solution which offers the best care to the most people will be implemented. Thus, I conclude using the Law of Large numbers that Telemedicine is the "average solution" and the way most Chinese seniors will receive geriatric care in the future. What's more, Telemedicine and a senior living facility are not mutually exclusive. Even those seniors living in

---

22 These all come from Johnathan D. Linkous, CEO of ATA

China's new assisted living facilities could avail themselves of this technology and facility operators can, thereby, increase their revenue while decreasing their fixed costs.

There is yet another reason to expect a Telemedicine "average" solution or outcome. China, over the past 30 years has taken large leaps and bypassed certain technology waypoints in their route to further modernization and "Mu Bai realities". Witness, the land line telephone: the West used land line telephones for 40 years before cellular technology was developed. But because of China's emergence onto the global scene relatively late last century there was no need for widespread use of land line telephone technology. Essentially, China jumped immediately to cellular phones and skipped a whole generation of communications technology. After all, cellular communications was less expensive, more effective and easier to implement across a vast geographic region. Telemedicine should be no different. This example is just further support for the thesis of this essay that Telemedicine is the future not just of health care in China, but of geriatric medicine especially.[23]

Once China internalizes the fiscal constraints of traditional, "Westernized" senior care for its burgeoning elderly population, discharges the obsession with historical geriatric care programs as well as its fixation on "branding", it will "let go" and achieve the "Mu Bai reality" of Telemedicine. This technology will enable modern, geriatric care for tens of millions of Chinese seniors in far flung locations, inexpensively and in a way that retains their independence. None of this is to say that Western geriatric care competencies are not highly appropriate to a China application. In fact they are, and significant export opportunity exists here

---

23 Of course, certain health care issues such as dementia don't really work well under a telemedicine application. But there are devices that can monitor patient wandering very effectively and unobtrusively.

for Western practitioners in so long as these skills are "trans-culturated" and delivered in a Chinese context; in doing so an ironic twist of circumstances might occur and the West may also achieve the "Mu Bai reality" of Telemedicine.

Technology solutions are product dependent. Banks could not roll out the Automated Teller Machine revolution until a manufacturer crafted and created the ATM product for the banks to deploy. The Chinese are marvelously adept at developing new products and then manufacturing them with remarkable quality and efficiency. Thus, there is a product challenge hidden within the technology response as the geriatric population burgeons and the need for responsive services explodes. A hidden opportunity lurks with Telemedicine and it is poised to leap like some striped feral beast!

As a final amusing and certainly less serious thought, I can envision an appropriate sequel to <u>Crouching Tiger, Hidden Dragon</u> *which might contain further dialogue between Mu Bai and Shu Lien, now in their 80's and elderly themselves, as follows:*

Mu Bai, now pre-diabetic, has just completed his blood pressure analysis and his glucose test. He presses the green send button to transfer his data to the central assessment unit. He looks up at Shu Lien, who having just finished her own self-assessment with their State provided Telemedicine monitor, is preparing for a session of morning Tai Chi with co-stars Jen, Lo and Sir Te.

Mu Bai sits back in his chair and says to Shu Lien: "Shu Lien, although I am no longer as agile as I was so many years ago, but I would like to go back to Wudan Mountain for further meditation.... come with me Shu!"

Shu Lien, also still young at heart but often forgetful replies: "Mu, please leave these things to the young warriors. We have mahjong after lunch and....I don't remember....but our afternoon is busy!"

Mu Bai insists: "Dutiful wife! My Telemedicine device is portable! We are going!" Mu Bai begins to stand quickly but his ageing knees force him back to his seat.

Shu, coming to help Mu Bai stand, reassures him: "Dear husband, let us be grateful for our independent lifestyle and accept this new, harmonious living for aged persons........Mu Bai, it has a permanence that is indeed real."

Camera fades to nearby Wudan Mountain.

Intermission: The Healthy Green Tea of Hangzhou
中场片段: 杭州健康绿茶

Moutai is to Guizhou what Longjing tea, or Dragon Well tea as its name is known in Mandarin, is to Zhejiang province. The tea is slightly bitter but it isn't enough to turn me away, in fact I like the coppery taste and it is so very Chinese. If you like Longjing tea, you will love Hangzhou as there are rivers of this tea there.

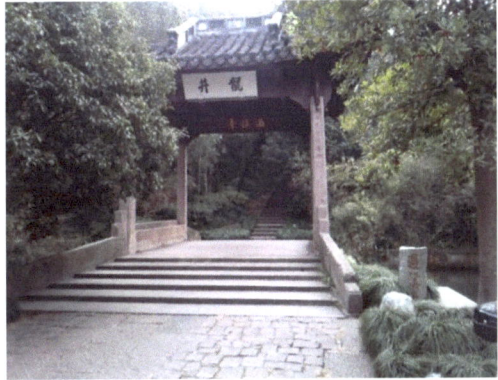

Figure 9 A longjing tea plantation in Hangzhou

As tea histories go, Longjing has a story which only could have been acquired in China. I imagine India has equally colorful stories about their tea, I don't know; but Longjing certainly has a colorful one. According to many reports, the tea was granted the status of Gong Cha, or Imperial tea, in the Qing Dynasty by Emperor Kangxi.[24] According to the legend, the illustrious Qing Emperor Kangxi's grandson, Qianlong (name means "Lasting Eminence")[25] visited Hangzhou's West Lake during one of his famous holidays laboring with his courtesans. He went to the Hu Gong Temple near the Lion Peak Mountain (Shi Feng Shan) and was presented with a cup of Longjing tea as he sat in front of the temple. Emperor-in-waiting Qianlong was so impressed by the Longjing tea produced in Hangzhou that he conferred upon the 18 tea trees that grew in front of the temple a special imperial status, afterwards endorsed

24 Emperor Kangxi 1654-1722, one of China's greatest leaders, oversaw a period of great calm, artistic achievement and wealth.

25 Lived 1722–1799. He was the sixth emperor of the Manchu-led Qing Dynasty, and the fourth Qing emperor to rule over China proper. Qianlong furthered Kangxi's efforts and brought enduring prosperity to the Qing.

by Kangxi. The trees are still living and the tea they produce is auctioned annually for more money per gram than gold.

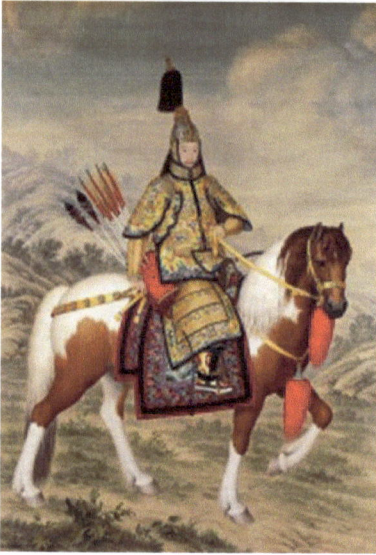

Figure 10 Qianlong – as painted by Guiseppe Castiglione 1758 (Wkpd)

But you should drink Longjing tea, not because Qianlong loved it or that his trees produce very expensive Longjing, but because it contains very high quantities of vitamin C, amino acids and most importantly, huge amounts of catechins. The health benefits of catechins, a type of antioxidant also found in red wine and chocolate albeit in lesser amounts, have been studied extensively in humans and animals. These amazing little molecules reduce artery plaque, carcinogens, the prevalence of stroke and diabetes.[26]

Qianlong lived to 77 a very old man for the 18th century; no doubt the healthy effect of Hangzhou's Longjing tea in abundance.

26 Norman Hollenberg, professor of medicine at Harvard Medical School, 1999.

Mao's Last Nursing Home
毛 时 代 最 后 的 敬 老 院

"The inherent vice of capitalism is the unequal sharing of blessings; the inherent virtue of communism is the equal sharing of miseries".
Winston Churchill

同 志 们 好! There is a nursing home in Wuxi called Liang Xiao (name changed). It is located down a side alley off a busy street not far from the central train station. Like most Starlight program acute care facilities in China, it is a grey and depressing place with little apparent security and wholly inadequate patient supervision. I don't know when Liang Xiao was built and the distressed nature of the buildings offer little clue; as most public facilities (with the notable exception of important government offices) are poorly constructed, it could just as easily be 10 years old as it could 30 years old. In all, Liang Xiao seems as hopeless and miserable a place as are its despondent and forlorn patients; fragility seems the least of their ailments as patient quality of life is non-existent. To be fair though, Liang Xiao did have an uncommon amount of activity and the type of motion that suggests design; but it wasn't clear at the time just what it was all about. Like most acute care geriatric facilities in China, it is over capacity by at least 10%.

I was invited to visit Liang Xiao as a result of one of their nurses having read information my firm, Hampton Hoerter China, was posting onto Weibo, the Chinese Twitter. We arranged our visit and scheduled the trip for an early afternoon arrival. Our hosts were the doctors and nurses who run the facility and we were told, the Chairman of the company. This last bit of information was curious as I was under the impression that all Starlight nursing homes were owned by the state. The purpose of our invitation was to learn if there was any opportunity for us to consult and assist Liang Xiao with their interest in upgrading their geriatric care program.

Shortly after our arrival and once done with the ceremonial exchange of business cards, fanfare of good wishes, obligatory sip of tea and taste of fruit, we were offered a tour of Liang Xiao which we graciously accepted and were told that Chairman Chang would be slightly delayed. And sure enough, twenty minutes into our tour the Chairman arrived with an entourage of 6 men attending to his calls, carrying his 3 briefcases and just generally making a scene about his arrival. Clearly, the intended impression to be conveyed by this activity was that Chairman Chang was exceedingly important and a much too busy person with whom to be trifled. Our tour guide noticed the Chairman's entrance and nervously diverted us from our route to the courtyard in the center of Liang Xiao where a brief introduction was to be made and photos taken. Chairman Chang was given our brochure by one of his assistants and as he read it out loud, he shook each of our hands. Once the introduction was complete, the Chairman insisted that our tour be postponed until later that afternoon and we should all, at once, retire to the luncheon which had been especially prepared for us.

Our lunch cleared up the mystery of the Chairman as well as Liang Xiao's noticeable bustle and opened a door of perception into what might well be the future of nursing homes in China. Calling the Chairman a businessman is a profound understatement, as he is more aptly described as one of China's new generation of ravenous entrepreneurs, a new breed of savvy and sharp-eyed capitalists who can spot opportunity a mile away; a man with a hundred wives to be sure. The Chairman's story begins a couple of years ago when the 12th 5 year plan was being written and the government began to allocate funds for the development of senior living facilities. Through what I can only imagine is a carefully constructed and meticulously maintained, salubrious network of political and business contacts (legendary guanxi) in Wuxi, Mr. Chang crafted himself an opportunity from the ruins of Liang Xiao. And while Mr. Chang doesn't know a thing about nursing care or even the management of such a facility, we must always remember the 4th philosophy of the Joy Longevity Club….General Tsao's copycat chicken with tasty sauce. The Chairman has visited North America for the express purpose of learning all he can from the senior living industry.

Through grants available via the Ministry of Civil Affairs and more importantly private investment, Chairman Chang is slowly turning Liang Xiao around, and even though it may not look like that today, having been to many other nursing homes in China over the past two years, the Chairman is clearly on the power curve of his industry. What is even more curious is that Chairman Chang has also "purchased" shares in Liang Xiao and through his private company "owns" a substantial minority stake. I use the quotations for effect here the inner machinations enabling this or the details of the structure are unclear; like many things in China the means justify the end and it is likely all informally arranged between him and his local government friends. These particulars notwithstanding, it is the big picture that is the point here: the Chairman is moving an industry that has long been mired in China's dismal legacy of anemic public health care. Chairman Chang and those who come after him in Wuxi (not to mention the 39,545 other public nursing homes in China) will no doubt profit handsomely from their efforts and they should; theirs is truly a herculean task.

This all reminds me in a way of Li Cunxin's gripping autobiography Mao's Last Dancer (and subsequent film adaptation by Bruce Beresford in 2009). In his book, Li Cunxin is born into a poor family commune in a small rural village in Shandong Province, where he is destined to work in the fields as a laborer. At first overlooked but eventually selected after suggestion by his teacher during a school visit, Li seems bewildered by the gruff preliminary inspection screening at the province capitol

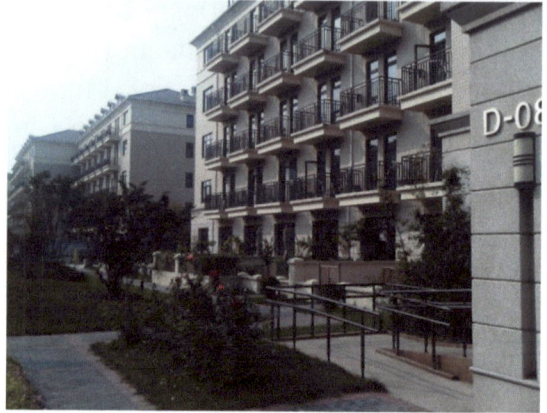

Figure 11 Sub-acute care building D-08 at General's Garden, Beijing

city of Qingdao. He is selected to travel to Beijing to audition for a place in Madame Mao's Dance Academy, and is admitted to its ballet school after passing a series of physical examinations. Years of arduous training follow, until his initial mediocre performance is finally overcome due to inspiration from a teacher's devotion to classical ballet as opposed to the politically motivated, strident form favored by Madame Mao. His determination and courage leads to him being grudgingly permitted by the Academy to travel abroad to Ben Stevenson's Houston Ballet company as a visiting student for three months. In the United States, he begins to question the Chinese Communist Party dictates upon which he has been raised, detaches himself from his political past, defects and flourishes as a dancer.

I see the Chairman as China's health care Li Cunxin; a charismatic, determined soul who sees more and desires a better circumstance for himself and his business and is frustrated with the status quo. The big difference between Li Cunxin and Chairman Chang is that the Chairman no longer has to defect to realize his ambition; China has learned to provide opportunities for those who are motivated enough.

A short injection of China's nursing home history

In 2000, China's Ministry of Civil Affairs announced the "Star Light (Xing Guang) Program" whereby the Ministry allocated 20% of the social welfare lottery fund to build community welfare facilities for seniors. From 2001 to 2004, the Chinese government invested a total of 13.4 billion yuan in this program and built 32,000+ "Star Light Centers for Seniors." The services of these centers are overly broad with multiple functions and cover family visits, emergency aid, day care, health care services, and recreational activities to over 30 million elders. At the same time, the government also increased its investment in building nursing homes to provide institutional care for older people in the "Star Light Program". Another program, the "Beloved Care Engineering" program began in 2005 and is aimed at increasing the number of nursing homes and encouraging good nursing home care quality through a government-sponsored Elder Care Foundation. These facilities range from senior citizens' lodging houses (apartments), older people homes, and nursing homes for the aged, which serve to meet elders with different functional abilities and financial backgrounds. The building of older people homes in rural areas was also encouraged for persons who can avail themselves of the "5 guarantees" which, when translated, are the basic needs of "food," "clothing," "accommodation," "health care," and "burial service". Those who can find their way into such accommodations are usually former revolutionary guards, government employees or other "proud" occupations. By the end of 2005, there were 39,546 institutions providing vastly different types of services for seniors with most providing subpar care, when compared with their Western counterparts (an admittedly unfair comparison). In total these institutions provided 1.497 million beds.

If providing nursing homes was the only issue then China would be well on her way, however that is the least of concerns. As with most endeavors on the mainland, human resources or lack thereof is usually the issue that trumps the best laid plans. The major source of health care workers are (often called "bao mu" in Chinese) laid-off workers in previously state-run factories, migrant workers from rural villages or unemployed ethnic minorities. They often do not have any training in elder care or nursing home care before they start working in the nursing homes for older adults. For laid-off workers, 1 to 2 days of short training in basic personal care is provided free of charge by some local government agencies, for example the Labor, Social Security Bureau, China Committee on Aging, and Women's Federation. However, none of these workers are required to have formal training in geriatric care before they enter into their work. As a result, the quality of care is grim and dangerously low. These workers are often required to pay a fee for these training courses and as this imposes a great financial difficulty, they usually do not enroll before they commence working. Such labor also presents other issues for working in nursing homes; different language or dialect, customs from those of urban cities' older people and cultural prejudices of patients who often dislike their care being given by "bao mu".[27]

As of April 2012, we hadn't yet begun our work with the Chairman, although I am confident we will do a great deal with him. And as you can imagine, the benefits of working with such a person extend far beyond simple contract remuneration. His highly choreographed performance to date in raising Liang Xiao from little more than a living graveyard to real, albeit Spartan, nursing home is nothing short of virtuosic.

---

27 This history of nursing homes, was drawn in near totality from "Nursing Homes in China" by Leung-Wing Chu, FRCP, and Iris Chi, MSW, DSW 2008

Intermission: Dalian Cepa Civitatem
中场片段: 大连层层叠

Generally, onions get a bad rap but some of their reputation is in fact deserved. Not only do they make you cry but they are awfully complex vegetables with so many layers. Peel away hundreds of translucent coatings in search of that which is the essence of onion, and one ultimately finds tearful disappointment; there is no core, no conclusion or an insignificant one at best. The inescapable finale, taste and utility notwithstanding: onions obfuscate, tease and frustrate. If only the onion diffused patience or perseverance instead of that lachrymatory agent, syn-propanethial-S-oxide, it might atone for its unscrupulous ways. Alas, the onion shows no such mercy; more a cunning approach is required to outwit this vegetable's treachery.

There was once a deal to be had in the City of Dalian, China. A tall building of 60 stories stands finished, but for upper floor fenestration and interior fit-out, in the center city. The previous owner, a Hong Kong developer, ran aground financially in the late 1990's and hadn't any more funds to complete the project. The 5 Chinese banks who had participated in the lending spree to finance this development seized control of the premises in 2004. The Chinese authorities take a dim view of bankruptcy, even a forced one, but that was the only option at hand to rid themselves of the borrower. Since then the building has languished, frequent looting has stripped the vacant building of much of its plumbing and squatters are invading. If the project isn't completed soon, thereby protecting the bank's investment, the building will need to be razed.

In 2009, a Korean businessman reached out to Dalian city officials and offered a deal to the city and the banks: his strategy – to purchase the debt, take control of the project, finish construction and sell the units off...making onion soup out of onions, one might say. After all, many investors have done quite well fixing the mistakes of others; distressed investing is not unknown to the Chinese. Yet the weakness in the Korean's plan was that he didn't know just how many layers this Dalian onion contained nor, as it turns out, was he prepared for such a complex endeavor.

Indeed, a brief investigation of the opportunity revealed layer upon layer of city approvals would be required, more consideration, endorsements and permissions from banks and yet still further agreements would be necessary from 4 separate courts to finalize disposition. To add to the complexity, any foreign investment in the project would require what is known as a WOFE[28] structure and approval from MOFCOM[29], all of which add more layers of work each entailing its own series of separate authorizations. After so much

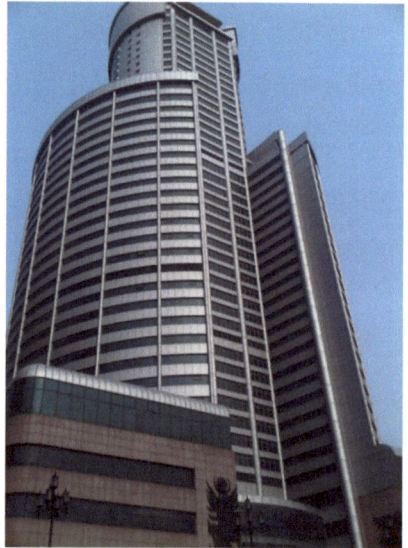

Figure 12 A unfinished, multi-purpose building in downtown Dalian

paring back of issues, the core of the project became visible; and how disillusioning it was. It was discovered that residential investment in China by foreign capital was to be placed on hold; the Dalian onion had reduced the Korean businessman to a sobbing wreck. He lost his deposits and since returned home to Seoul.

---

28 Wholly owned foreign entity – the vehicle often used by foreigners to invest in China.

29 Ministry of Commerce of the People's Republic of China.

A sharp blade is a handy item when it comes to onions; slicing neatly through so many layers limits cell damage and reduces the release of enzymes that force tearing. Likewise developing Chinese-like business acumen to quickly penetrate complex municipal structures, deliberate obstructions, and neatly carve through red tape for red tape sake without getting consumed with details or running afoul of local customs is a necessary quality that the Korean could have used to avoid this sad end.

A final note: There are a lot of onions in China, not just in Dalian. In fact it is world's largest onion grower having produced 20.5 million metric tons of the vegetable in 2012.

Farewell my Migrant Health Care Worker
告 别 了 流 动 护 理 工 时 代

"A smile ushers in the Spring and a tear does darken all the world",
*Master Yuan in **Farewell my Concubine***

同 志 们 好! What follows below is a slightly edited transcript of an interview with a young woman named "Jiang" (alias) which occurred in Beijing, Chaoyang District at a Starbucks coffee shop on December 1, 2011. All edits are primarily due to issues of translation, my imperfect "on the run" typing effort and a very uncomfortable seat at Starbucks. Otherwise, her responses are reported below in as true a form as possible. The purpose of the interview is to shed light on the single most critical issue within the burgeoning geriatric care industry in China: namely, the absolute dearth of properly trained human resources and consequently the use of inadequately trained personnel to administer care to the elderly Chinese. A read through the interview illuminates other social concerns, and while I am sympathetic to these, my focus here is senior care.

Jiang is a young lady of 36 years who is a migrant health care worker in Beijing. She is perfectly average for her social cohort in nearly every respect: neither pretty nor ugly, simply dressed, with serious tooth decay and a limited world view. She is a contract employee at a state run nursing facility and has no professional education in nursing other than what she has learned over the past few years. Jiang, and many of the people with whom she works are known as "Bao Mu", or migrant workers. Being Bao Mu carries a stigma and it is not a pleasant one; they are viewed as wholly inferior, as a lower caste, dirty and unworthy. Bao Mu are usually ethnic minorities and they have largely been disenfranchised from the Chinese economic miracle. In reality, I found in Jiang bucolic charm and a meek honesty which set her in sharp contradiction to her current urban existence; indeed, to her, life in Beijing could not be more uncomfortably foreign.

As we moved through the discussion, Jiang became more relaxed and began to open up. I did not intend to enter the realm of her private life but as the interview progressed, it became obvious that her past has had profound influence on her current situation. Some of her answers are startling and painful; they paint a vivid picture of not only her job but of her life as well. Lastly, you will notice that the conversation is occasionally peppered with anecdotal comments, either before or after a question, in << >> brackets. I added these notes after a final proof read as I found a simple rote reproduction of the interview resulted in a hollowness which failed to sufficiently convey the emotional environment.

Jiang arrived at Starbucks prior to the translator and me. She was sitting at a small table in the back of the room waiting patiently with her coat and gloves on, giving a guarded impression that she considered us a potential no-show. As we approached the table she stood, smiled and said hello. After a brief introduction by the translator and some explanation, I began the interview:

Bromme 柯博明: Hello, Jiang.

Jiang: Hello Sir.

Bromme 柯博明: My name is 柯博明 and I have a business here in China. I help Chinese businesses build private nursing homes and senior living facilities. I have explained to you that I want to ask you a number of questions about the work you do, how you came to do it, what you think about it and generally about what you want to do in the future. Is this ok? You understand?

Jiang: Yes Sir.

Bromme 柯博明: Also, I am asking you these questions because I intend to publish your answers on a website I own and eventually include them in a book. You will remain anonymous, but your responses will be reproduced, after translation and small edits, in their entirety. This is ok for you?

Jiang: Yes Sir.

<<Jiang nods in approval>>

Bromme 柯博明: Ok, let's get started. Where were you born and where did you grow up?

Jiang: I was born in Bishan...I grew up there too; my entire life.

<<Bishan is a rural town near Chongqing. Jiang, obedient and dutiful, asks if she can take her coat off.>>

Bromme 柯博明: How old are you?

Jiang: 36

<<*She honestly looked much, much older...I was guessing 45*>>

Bromme 柯博明: How many years of education do you have? And what have you studied?

Jiang: I studied the basic curriculum.

<<*This means that Jiang spent nine years in school*>>

Bromme 柯博明： Jiang, I understand that you work in a nursing home, how long have you worked there?

Jiang: About three years…

Bromme 柯博明： What do you like most about it?

Jiang: The money, but I do not get paid much.

Bromme 柯博明： How much are you paid?

<<Glancing between the translator and me, Jiang was not eager to discuss her salary and I think she found this a little intrusive. There was some conversation between them about my question between the time I asked it and her final response. It was awkward for her and, I sensed a little painful. But I believe she was truthful.>>

Jiang: They pay me 1,500 RmB per month. I also get a bed and some food.

<<This equates to roughly USD235 plus the food and bed.>>

Bromme 柯博明： What do you like least about it?

Jiang: I do not like taking care of old people; I am a young person. The old people yell at me and sometimes try and hit me when I have to touch them.

Bromme 柯博明： Do you get hit a lot? Why do you have to touch them? What do you mean?

Jiang: Sometimes I get hit but often they miss me because they are slow. The nurses tell me I have to clean them when they shit in the bed. Or sometimes I have to help them go to the bathroom by inserting my finger into their anus. Also, sometimes the families blame us when the old people die.

<<*Jiang tried to release this bit of information as if she were sorting laundry, but she could not contain the anguish; it was embarrassing for her.*>>

Bromme 柯博明: Does anyone else hit you? Have the nurses every hit you? The boss?

Jiang: No. My father used to hit me but not the nurses.

<<*I choked on my breath. Obviously, this was unexpected and the result of a miscue in translation. It made both the translator and me a little uncomfortable, and I decided to ignore it for the time being. After a breath, I continued.*>>

Bromme 柯博明: How did you find your job here at the nursing home?

Jiang: My friends told me.

Bromme 柯博明: How did they find this job?

Jiang: I don't know.

Bromme 柯博明: What did you do before you worked at the nursing home?

Jiang: I was a food worker. I prepared food in a factory.

<<Her answers here were robotic and truly conveyed that she was disconnected to her job; it was merely a means to an end.>>

Bromme 柯博明: Jiang, when you left the factory (Where was the factory?) and came here to Beijing to work at the nursing home, what training did they give you?

Jiang: I worked in Wenzhou. When I was contracted, the nurses told me what to do and after a few weeks I was able to do most of the work alone.

<<Wenzhou is located on the coast of China, not far south of Shanghai. Wenzhou is the crucible of Chinese entrepreneurship.>>

Bromme 柯博明: And today, do you work unsupervised?

Jiang: Yes, most of the day.

Bromme 柯博明: Other than clean the patients, what else are your duties?

Jiang: I feed them, give them medicine, help wash them, help them exercise if they want.

Bromme 柯博明: Jiang, how long do you think you will work at the nursing home? Do you have other plans? What would you like to do with your life after the nursing home?

<<This question was either puzzling to Jiang or the translation was off. It took a few iterations to get it on target>>

Jiang: I have to work here because I need the money. Someday I might find another job but I don't know. I would like not to work here, but I don't know where to go. I would like to have a shop and sell things.

Bromme 柯博明: What type of things would you like to sell?

Jiang: All sorts of things, cute little knickknacks, dolls, sweets!

<<Jiang turned into a little girl describing this. She was almost excited and literally disappeared into another world for a moment.>>

Bromme 柯博明: So, Jiang, if I understand you correctly, you work at the nursing home for no other reason than you need the money? Right? You essentially hate the job, nothing about it interests you. In fact, caring for the old people disgusts you...they even hit you sometimes, right?

Jiang: Yes Sir.

Bromme 柯博明: Do you think you are good at your job? Are you proud to be a health care worker?

Jiang: Today I know my job and I do it, but I do not like it. I am not proud of being a health care worker...it is a low job.

<<The idea of being proud of her job was novel, but once she understood the question, she responded with little hesitation>>

Bromme 柯博明: Do you think being a health care worker is an important job?

Jiang: It is not an important job, if it were I would be paid more money.

<<Jiang's logic was unassailable and her honesty was simple. I was beginning to sense that this idea of mine, that is to interview a migrant health care worker, needed something more. So I decided on a different track>>

Bromme 柯博明: I want to ask you some questions not related to your job at the nursing home, ok?

Jiang: Yes.

Bromme 柯博明: Did you have a happy childhood and are your parents still alive?

<<I felt this was a reasonable subject to explore given her prior admission about her father.>>

Jiang: My parents are alive. We are a very poor family. And when I was little my parents had to split up and work in different cities. I had to go and live with my relatives for a long time. One day my father came to get me and take me home. But he would beat me all day and tell me to call my mother and beg her to come home. I had a very bad relationship with my father.

<<Jiang opened up here in a way that I doubt she has in quite some time. She was almost eager to say these things. Her answer above is an abridged version of her entire response.>>

Bromme 柯博明: If you could buy anything what would it be?

Jiang: A nice house for my mother and a shop for me!

<<Jiang smiled broadly. She missed her mother enormously>>

Bromme 柯博明: Jiang, I have only a few more questions. When your mother is old and frail will you take care of her? Or would you consider a nursing home for her?

Jiang: Yes, I will care for her.

<<Jiang oozed empathy>>

Bromme 柯博明: But you will have to work, right? How will you take care of her and work at the same time?

Jiang: I don't know.

<<And again, Jiang's honesty was never more apparent than in this answer. She paused for a while before answering, looked down at the floor hopelessly and responded without looking up. I think that this may have been the first time she ever considered the difficult situation of either caring for the mother she loves more than anything or supporting herself. I don't want to read too much into her answer but I suspect that she began to rethink her plight at this moment. Her answer in a way almost made me feel guilty about presenting her with this dilemma>>

Bromme 柯博明: Jiang, do you have any questions for me?

Jiang: Sir, why do you want to work in nursing homes?

<<Clever girl, I thought>>

Bromme 柯博明: I don't really work in them. I help people build them and operate them.

<<Jiang waited for the translation. It didn't appear that my response really answered her question.>>

Bromme 柯博明: Thank you, Jiang. I have enjoyed speaking with you.

Jiang: Yes Sir. Did I do a good job?

Bromme 柯博明: Yes, Jiang. You did a great job.

<<Jiang rose from the table and put her jacket back on. She thanked the translator, smiled and began to walk out, when I asked her one last question>>

Bromme 柯博明: Oh, ah…Jiang..?

Jiang: Yes Sir?

<<Jiang pauses and turns to look at me…she smiles broadly>>

Bromme 柯博明: Have you ever seen the Chinese movie *Farewell My Concubine*?

Jiang: Oh, no Sir, I don't know what that is. Anyway movies are too expensive. Goodbye!

Bromme 柯博明: Goodbye, Jiang.

<<Jiang turned and walked towards the exit. For all the weight she carried on her small shoulders, she had a carefree bounce in her step as she slid through the glass doors and waved one last time.>>

In my two hours with her, I found Jiang to be much like Chen Dieyi in the film *Farewell my Concubine.* Not on a superficial level, but in terms of how tortured she must be; caught in the middle of a miserable triangle with the angles of her life defined by a father who beat her as a child, the necessity of holding down a job she despises and a mother to whom she is fully devoted and loves dearly but cannot live with for financial reasons. Making this mosaic more complex, Jiang knows that she, like millions of other

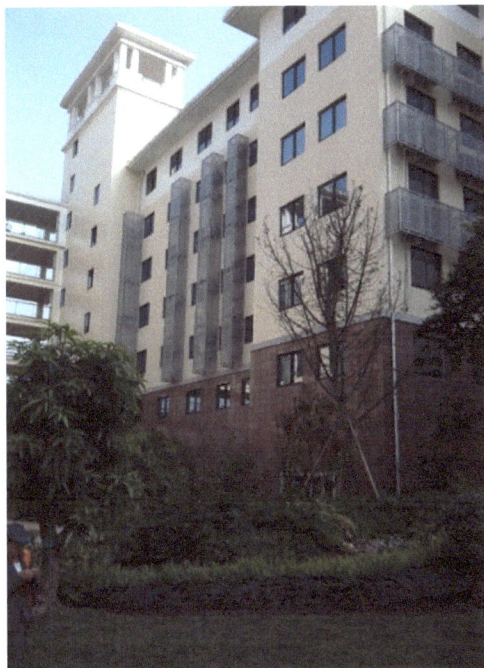

Figure 13 Qinggang Elderly Nursing Center: 1st Affiliated Hospital of Chongqing

poor and middle income Chinese, face a dreadful dilemma of ultimately having to care for their parents and lose a job or keep the job and turn their parents over to a nursing home. This dynamic is one reason for the decline of traditional filial piety in China and its evolution into something more modern that will make facility living an acceptable option.

Update: Last week I found myself in the vicinity of the nursing home where Jiang works. I stopped by to say hello and thank her again for her time. The manager of the facility seemed frustrated when I inquired about her; he told me she had quit her job three days ago and did not know where she went.

She just left he explained, raising his hands in exasperation, "Like all the Bao Mu, appear from nowhere and disappear into nowhere".

I turned and walked out of the nursing home, leaving behind the caustic tang of bleach and sour reek of dirty clothes. The cold air bit into my nose and cleared my lungs as I stepped outside. I walked down the street and thought about what the manager said regarding Bao Mu disappearing into nowhere. As I hailed

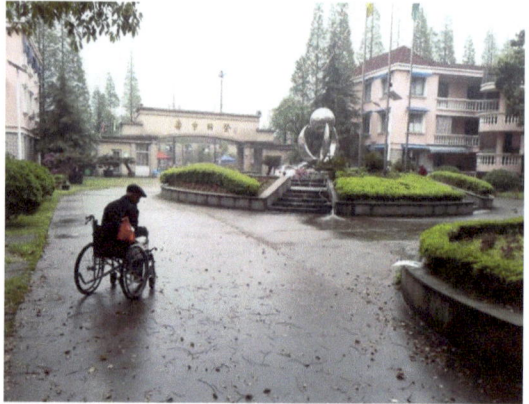

Figure 14 Red Maple Senior living facility in Wenzhou; one of China's earliest...built in 1992

a cab, I looked back at the nursing home and imagined Jiang, an apparition with suitcase in hand, furtively leaving her job, escaping under the cover of a foggy dawn.

Full of ephemeral sympathy for Jiang, I thought to myself as I got into the cab, "Indeed...'*disappearing into nowhere*,'...has there ever been a more poignant, unknown destination?"

Intermission: Impermanent Shenzhen!
中场片段: 深圳漂移

I've been to this City five times in the past 3 years and it never has been the same, except for the border crossing...the same building, the same guards... that fixed, immovable point of departure before one leaves the realm of certainty and enters a world of transience; welcome to Shenzhen. A City born

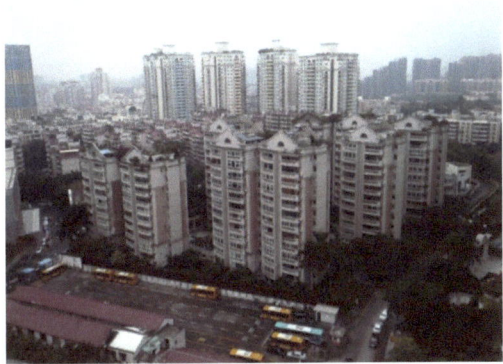

Figure 15 View of Hua Qiao Cheng, Shenzhen

into existence in the 1980's as part of Deng Xiao Peng's economic experiment with a capitalist future; where all things were intended to be temporary, always undergoing further improvement yet never complete, where durability became synonymous with obsolescence. In Shenzhen, the temporal nature of life is tangible; buildings are torn down daily and rebuilt in months, new roads are planned, ploughed and paved overnight, and neighbors are replaced with the seasons. In fact, the city's demonym "Shenzhener" could be a synonym for passenger.

Most cities require effort to know and offer rewarding memories to those who search, inquire and pry. The Shenzhen experience offers no such prize; no distracting historical sites, no imposing cultural attractions...just an incessant stream of modern consumption for the here and now with an acquisitive eye winking at tomorrow. Here there are no citizens only 10.3 million transients swept up in an undertow of material obsession who then disappear into a sea of anonymity. In Shenzhen personal relationships are kept to a minimum; people come and go speaking only of their portfolios. There is no other city like it in the world.

Shenzhen is mercilessly commercial and for its purpose this may or may not be a good thing. In a way it is a modern counterpart to the 1930 company towns in the US which gave questionable refuge to destitute sharecropper families. As is true, more poignantly, of Shenzhen's Foxconn mini-city; a hive of humanity swarming with those who have escaped the extreme poverty of rural China only to realize the Orwellian existence of assembly-line life. In Shenzhen there is a deep Chinese ethnographic and cultural anthropologic narrative unfolding. A profound Chinese tale on the level of Agee's *Now let us praise famous men* waits to be written about this City. But such a deep, introspective inquiry is unlikely to be written by a local. Despite its reputation as one of China's most liberal cities, Shenzhen is still part of China and therefore will likely tolerate no substantive, self-critical biography for some time; alas, even for the city that changes every day, something remains the same.

Impermanence, or Wuchang in Mandarin, expresses the Buddhist notion that all of existence, without exception, is in a constant state of flux, always changing; forever mutable and endlessly fluid. Indeed, Shenzhen...the Wuchang city...she wakes up each day a new city with no history only future.

All Aboard!......This is the China CCRC Express!
到点了！上车啦！.....长者颐养特快列车！

同 志 们 好! "It took more than one man to change my name to Shanghai Lily," purrs Marlene Dietrich in Josef von Sternberg's film 1932 adaptation of Harry Hervey's book *Shanghai Express*. She certainly has her well-manicured talons sunk into more men than she can count in this exotic far-Eastern, chiaroscuro-cinematographic adventure. Among her fellow passengers on the Shanghai Express are her disenchanted former fiancé, unshakable British medical officer Clive Brook; over-zealous missionary Lawrence Grant; dope smuggler Gustav von Seyffertitz; and enigmatic Eurasian businessman Warner Oland. Coincidently, Oland made frequent appearances in other China-themed movies, most notably as Charlie Chan, the benevolent and heroic Chinese detective based in Honolulu.

As the train chugs through the more treacherous passages of war-torn China, Oland reveals himself as the leader of a rebel group, who plans to hold the passengers hostage to secure the release of his imprisoned constituents. In Boule de Suif fashion, Dietrich, who portrays a notorious "Chinese coaster" has remained sexually remote throughout the trip, gives herself to Oland to save the life of Brook, the man she truly loves. Directed by Josef von Sternberg at his most orgiastic (check out the long, lingering dissolves!), and unlike this essay, *Shanghai Express* is 80% style and 20% substance.

Tickets, *please*....

This essay is about China's 3 largest and most visible geriatric care developments to date. I warn you in advance, it is also my longest essay yet but the information conveyed is important for those interested in senior living in China. Each of these projects has been in the market for at least 2 years and in one case nearly 5 years. I call them CCRC's (continuing care retirement communities) because, well, that is what they set out to be and in some part that is what the developers have accomplished...or, better yet, are clearly struggling to accomplish. One of these developments had the benefit of limited foreign assistance, the others did not. The one that did clearly benefited and consequently has the best aged-care program in China today. All are chugging along with common weaknesses and each has their strengths. In sum, it is a mixed bag and to the inexperienced eye (read: China senior living experience, not western senior living experience; I say this as nearly all western geriatric care practitioners who see their first China project immediately conclude that all China senior care is a train wreck) it might seem as if the idea of senior living in China is just on the wrong track. But it is early and the train hasn't left the station, at least not just yet.

Those who seek to conduct the senior care business in China are well advised to remember a few important rules of the China elder care experience: first, China senior living is where Western geriatric care was in 1950 but gathering steam quickly; second, never judge a project out of context, meaning: comparing a project in Chongqing to a project in Santa Barbara is meaningless as the buyers of the Chongqing project don't have that choice much less that perspective; third, the higher one stays in the acuity chain, the more leverage one has...which translates into success; and finally, for the time being, stay in the high-end or 1st class coach, period.

Before this train departs, I would like to make one last observation. My thoughts below are a mildly critical analysis bordering on subjective evaluation and at times, some literary lampooning. Lest I be detained by the People's Senior Living Police at Beijing Nan Zhan (FYI: an enormous train station), I beg merciful consideration that these contemplations be seen not as cruel condemnation, malicious denigration, negative commentary or, heaven forbid, Confucian blasphemy of any CCRC discussed here or China's senior living potential in general. Quite the contrary, I am no apostate; I see a bright future and if these three communities are indications of what the Chinese can accomplish right out of the box, then the next decade will be outstanding for professionals in the China geriatric care business.

And finally, as the whistle blows, for those readers not entirely familiar with a CCRC, they are usually defined as a campus style residential complex assembling a market driven mix of 1) independent living residences (IL) for active but senior adults, 2) assisted living units (AL) for older adults needing some support with their daily activities and 3) skilled nursing care for frail or infirm adults requiring frequent assistance or acute medical care. Additionally, there are often a variety of cultural amenities, exercise facilities and commercial support services which offer basic necessities and provisions, such as hair salon, laundry/dry cleaners and variety store.

First stop, General's Garden.....*General's Garden!*

When I first visited General's Garden nearly two years ago, I thought, "This is it....modern senior living has indeed arrived in China". But after my fourth trip and some pretty rigorous investigation and analysis, I began to see the cracks in both hardware and software. In a sense, the General's Garden's locomotive was running out of steam.

General's Garden was opened to the public around 2009. It is located in the northeast quadrant of Beijing (off 4th ring road), not far from Beijing Capital International airport and the Museum of

Film. The land was Ministry of Transport land and the property's perimeter remains a testing track for China's high-speed railway. I refer to General's Garden as a CCRC as it loosely embodies a simple definition of a CCRC, as outlined above. Indeed, General's Garden offers 51 villas or large townhouse style residences with private gardens, 280+ independent/assisted living apartments and 160 skilled nursing units all within a gated compound. This facility also offers a 3-hole golf course (plus driving range), an unusual, man-made forested park, an unfeasibly large and as of yet unfinished 17,000m² hot-spring clubhouse, an 160 room inn for visitors and a clinic specializing in traditional Chinese medicine.

So what happened? Well, as of January 2012, only 14 of the Villas had sold and less than 10 residents purchased golf course memberships (which by the way, through October of last year, boasted an expensive, resident Australian PGA Pro to give lessons to all those resident members). I would get into detail about the amenity membership program but it is way too complicated (e.g. Golf course membership is priced on ball usage). The villas ranging in size from 700-800 square meters, carry a price tag of between RmB

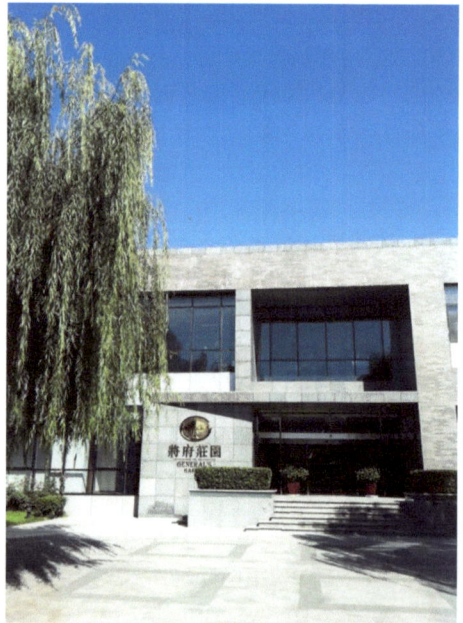

Figure 16 Entrance to General's Garden, Beijing

45 million and RmB 55 million for unfinished space and the IL/AL units go for RmB 1.5 million plus services on an as needed,

menu basis. And while the IL/AL living apartments and the skilled nursing units are fairly well occupied (75%-80%), there are likely a number of reasons for the stalled performance of the villas. As an aside, I have to note that the best thing about General's Garden is the aged-care program; it was set up by an Australian group and they did a superlative job. Until recently, an Australian also continued to manage this section of the facility; he has a great deal of experience and insight into how Chinese seniors need/want geriatric care. Kudos to this master of the China senior care experience! Our access to General's Garden's business plan has allowed us to tabulate much of their rental and sales data which we share with clients.

Unlike the Little Engine That Could, (*"I think I can, I think I can..."*) the General's Garden villas have never made it up the hill. I believe this is because: 1) the land on which the facility is built is known as "collective land" which does not convey fee title to the buyer, only a long term lease (approximately 50 years for either a villa or an IL/AL unit). Consequently, potential purchasers are faced with an unappealing opportunity to buy an enormously expensive, depreciating asset which under Chinese law cannot be hypothecated, 2) General's Garden never seemed to have a comprehensive marketing plan or buyer outreach program other than pursuing the ownership's network of political contacts for unit sales, and 3) perhaps the least understood aspect of the facility, its capitalization and financial game-plan which seemed, at best, *ad-hoc*. Beginning early last fall the warning signals were as subtle as a diesel engine's piercing whistle at 4am: contractors stopped receiving payments and construction stopped on the remaining units and clubhouse, there was a sharp increase in deferred maintenance, a hostile takeover occurred and subsequently, most senior management ceased receiving paychecks.

On the other hand the IL/AL units are, comparatively speaking, a success. And while ownership, meaning title conveyed, of such a unit is no different than that with a villa, they are much less expensive (in fact they are well priced at an average of RmB12,000m^2). It is interesting to note that there has been a trend of older adults buying these units for their children to live in…..however odd. Despite its raison d'être as a CCRC, no writ of Chinese law prevents young people from living there. I guess this is an indication of the facility's pricing as much as its attractiveness, or more likely, the parents intend to move in at some future date.

In late January 2012, new management at General's Garden, reeling from the enormity of their poorly analyzed, hostile acquisition, fired 12 persons many of whom were experienced senior managers. The terminal analysis is likely that General's Garden neglected to fully understand their market, didn't identify a target buyer and never adequately projected unit absorption against capital requirements to identify a breakeven point; a lethal mistake.

I will say though, in all fairness, this review of General's Garden must contain praise for the original management whose fundamental concept of this CCRC is a sound, well integrated facility; it is just the execution and some software that jumped the track. I have met the previous General Manager and those in his inner circle and believe he/they are talented people capable of positively impacting the senior living industry in China. His early efforts at the facility are proof of this and had it not been for the hostile take-over, General's Garden would continue to benefit from his leadership and likely turn the train around. However, without him General's Garden lacks vision and perspective; it faces a number of critical switches in the track ahead.

At this point, given the time of year in which this is being written[30], select a more solemn reference as a testament to this facility's narrative. With its fall from grace, perhaps we can call General's Garden and its story, "The Prodigal CCRC", a parable of squandered opportunity; now lost, can and better yet will, General's Garden atone for its marketing, repent its financial sins and find its way again?

Yanda....next stop...... *Yanda!*

Now this is a facility to behold. While its full name is a mouthful, Yanda Golden Age Health Nursing Center, the facility is frequently referred to as Yanda. One arrives at Yanda entering under an enormous, ceremonial gate and into a Tiananmen Square-like plaza large enough to park 500 tractor trailers. After

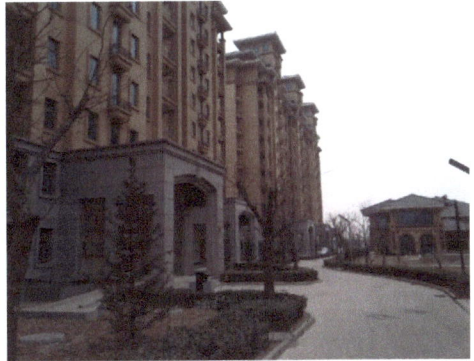

Figure 17 Yanda facility, Hebei Province

parking your car, walking around Yanda is, frankly, a little creepy and reminds me of the cities created in the narcotic-induced dreams of Dom Cobb in Christopher Nolan's *Inception*, ...beautiful, large, vacant and crumbling.

Yanda's first impediment is its location, situated a hard hour's drive from Chaoyang district, Beijing in adjacent Hebei province, it is tough to get too. Second, Yanda simply is overbuilt. So much of what has transpired at this facility is unclear, even the basic facts such as room count and beds are, in typical Chinese fashion,

---

30 Easter 2012

opaque. We are told there are 1,200 units at Yanda, but it feels like more. There is a 3,000 bed hospital (management claims 4 operations performed to date but most equipment remains shrink-wrapped) and a 200 bed geriatric nursing facility which, management professes is quite busy but there aren't a lot of cars in the parking lot and not a single ambulance arrived during my 3 hour tour (I arrived at lunch time). But hey, I won't let my lying eyes fool me, I saw not a single patient in the nursing care center. Wait…there is more: a 250+ room hotel and four places of worship (seriously): Buddhist, Muslim, Christian and Jesuit/Catholic all sited next to a bank (presumably for those whose faith favors Mammon). And if that isn't enough, ownership built a 30 story building that serves as living quarters for the health care workers who will, hopefully, arrive someday soon. Whew! What a budget!

Truly statuesque, in the lifeless sense of the word, this project should be renamed the "Colossus of Hebei" as colossal is the only term that adequately defines Yanda (well, maybe "stalled" has relevance here as well but lacks a certain visual onomatopoeia). Now, when confronted with the enigmatic and incomprehensible my imagination always runs wild. In fact, Yanda inspired in me a rewrite of those last few dreadful lines from the famous Shelley poem *Ozymandias*:

> "*....My name is Yanda, King of CCRC's: Look on my campus, ye mighty, and despair! Few residents remain. Round the decay of that colossal wreck, now budget-less and bare, the congested Chinese conurbation stretches far away*".

In all seriousness, here is the punch line: Yanda is only 20 percent occupied and it could well be less. I take this fact on face value from what we are told by the tour guide. But having been there at lunch, my favorite time to visit a facility as it reveals a lot, there certainly wasn't too much activity.

This is what we do know about Yanda: unlike General's Garden, Yanda is a pure rental scheme. Most occupants lease units on a year basis, but management also quotes 2 and 3 year options. Independent and assisted living units (1 and 2 bedrooms) rent for RmB 5,600 to RmB 9,600 per month plus services which can be selected from a menu. The nursing facility offers beds/units beginning at RmB 13,600 to RmB 16,800 per month, also depending on size and acuity. There is also another quirk to the pricing; the sponsor offers a kind of sinking fund whereby if you deposit sufficient monies with them, they will pay a 6% return on your money that is equal to your monthly rent (the number of takers for this generous offer is unknown). The young lady who showed me and my staff around, gave us the above 'rack rate" pricing (and a sheet with greater detail on it) but was eager to mention that we were very lucky customers and our visit today was auspicious; management has instructed her to offer high status individuals, such as ourselves, a one-time only, VIP discount of 40% on a full year lease for IL/AL units and a whopping 60% discount for nursing units. Days later, subsequent phones calls to verify information were met with the same offer.

Yanda opened up in 2010 and blew its steam before getting out of the station. The ROI has to be hurting by now and somebody is likely to take a loss going forward. It isn't an ugly project, in fact I found the basic design "ok" by China CCRC standards; but somebody has to take control of the marketing here, drive absorption aggressively and simplify the rental scheme before the buildings fall apart resolving the problem forever. This is the only prospect here: try and compete on price and program in an attempt to overcome Yanda's real weakness: location. Believe it or not, there is land allocated for a phase II....someday, hopefully never.

Cherish Yearn, last stop.......*everybody off!*

This facility's operations are as curious as its name. Located in a distant corner of Pudong, on a former duck farm, Cherish Yearn came to market about five years ago. It was an early arrival to the China senior living space and its organization, facility design and ambience all reflect its vintage. I first visited Cherish Yearn in late 2010 and quite honestly, I thought it was a disaster. From the dry and shriveled-up desert-like landscaping to the mold-stained stucco on the buildings; it had little ambience, few residents and zero energy.

Cherish Yearn was completed in 2006 and the first residents occupied in 2007. For years it struggled with occupancy and when I returned for a second visit in early 2012, I was pleasantly surprised. Apparently, over the past two years, a new marketing program was implemented and brought census up from a low of 20% to what is reported now as nearly 80%; and after my tour I believe the true figure is not far from this level. Activity rooms are busy with geriatric calligraphers; libraries are full of bespectacled Mandarins gazing over the Central Committee daily and even the computer rooms are full of elderly Chinese pecking away on keyboards. Indeed there is so much activity at Cherish Yearn its resurrection earns it a new name: the "Lazarus of Pudong"...so there is indeed hope for The Prodigal CCRC and the Colossus of Hebei.

Like its sister facilities, Cherish Yearn is large. It offers nearly 800+ units in 15 different mid-rise buildings. Independent living accounts for at least 600 units and there is a 300 bed nursing facility. The independent units have a reported 65% occupancy but it is entirely unclear how many residents are in the nursing facility. Access to the upper floors is prohibited but the first floor, which does indeed have patient rooms, reveals no activity whatsoever and is largely dark.

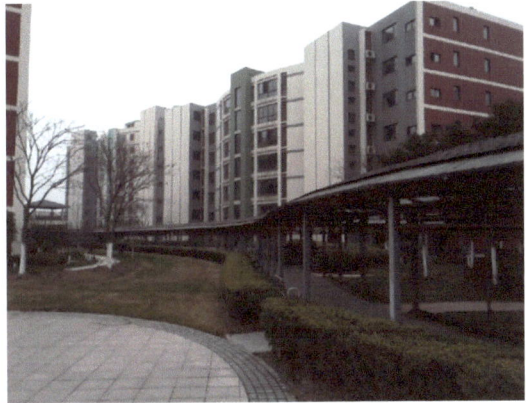

Figure 18 Cherish Yearn facility, Pudong Shanghai

Cherish Yearn's business model is founded on a membership scheme with an upfront fee and annual rental payments plus usage charges for the clubhouse and other amenities such as the dining hall. There are 2 basic plans: Plan A essentially confers title to the occupant for an entry fee of RmB 890,000. Once admitted, the resident may choose from 3 basic size units: large units ($108m^2$ or $1150ft^2$), medium units ($70m^2$ or $740ft^2$) and small units ($58m^2$ or $625ft^2$) each of which charges an annual fee according to size. A resident who has purchased a unit under Plan A may sell the unit himself at some future date or offer to the sponsor who will re-purchase it for 90% of the entry fee or market price, whichever is less. Plan B confers a 15 year right of use for an entry fee beginning at RmB 880,000 for a large unit, the smaller units have lower entry fees; there is also a static annual fee of RmB 29,800 across all unit types. Plan B's entry fee is refundable on a straight declining basis (calculated monthly) over the 15 year lease period.

Plan A seems to be most popular with children who wish to purchase a unit for their parents and Plan B seems to be the choice for elderly who buy for themselves. There are substantially more Plan B buyers than those who avail themselves of Plan A. We have completed a full tabular analysis of Cherish Yearn's fee structure which, again, is available to clients.

It is fair to mention that in the past, Cherish Yearn experienced some controversy over both its fundamental ability to offer sub-acute care services as well as its adherence to the original land grant use rights. The issues here may have been cleared up but there has been at least one published article in the media discussing the facility's "land rights" issue the details of which was supported by a credible, well connected source who has since spoken to me directly. In some quiet corners, rumors persist regarding the facility's legality, but in the end, I can see how this may just be envious chatter over Cherish Yearn's unprecedented success. Let's not forget, the truth in China has many layers.

So, in submissive genuflection, I offer faithful congratulations to the Lazarus of Pudong. Despite all, I believe it to be the most successful CCRC project today in China and its program is unique: truly a Chinese *sui generis* model.

The Terminus

Shanghai Lilly's assertion regarding the time and effort it took to secure her reputation whistles true and sharp about many endeavors in China; virtues such as patience and fortitude are essential. Likewise, it will take more than just a few attempts at CCRC development to perfect the model or models as the case is likely to be in China. CCRC's are complex undertakings and even in the West, developers with all their access to data and experience often misstep and build mistakes. So it is no surprise that the Chinese incarnation of a CCRC is a wobbly work in waiting. While I see near term success for the smaller, sub-acute facilities currently being built along the east coast of China by both foreign experts and local developers, nothing will dissuade, much less disabuse, the Chinese entrepreneur from pulling the heavy freight of a senior living mega-project. These immense CCRC's may be the track the industry ultimately takes. But for now, as of April 2013, CCRC's are not working in China and I think it will be 15 years before they catch on. For now, were I an investor or owner/operator, my concentration would remain focused on the light at the end of a tunnel: the more manageable, higher acuity, greater demanded and, say, narrow-gauge projects; let's call them the "Shanghai geriatric express".

Intermission: Welcome to Hohhot...Home of Glorious Mongu Peoples...Have a Nice Day!
中场片段: 欢迎来到呼和浩特… 蒙古人的家乡… 美好的一天

Population: 2.86 million
Founded: 1581 by Mongol ruler Altan Khan
Area: Capital of Inner Mongolia Autonomous Region
Location: 40°49'N 111° 39'E

On December 3, 2011 around 3:15pm Central China time, China Air flight 137 lowered its landing gear and sank below 2,000 feet. It was

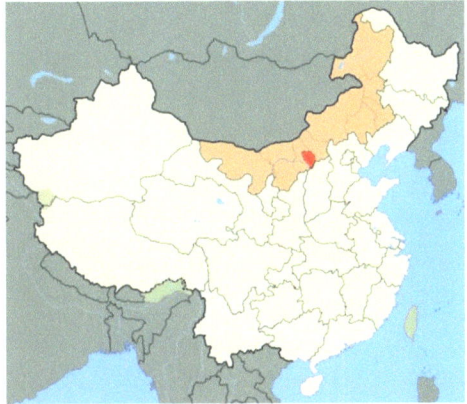

Figure 19 Inner Mongolia (orange) Hohhot (red) (Wkpd)

to be the last 15 minutes of a 13 hour flight which originated in New York's JFK airport. Looking out the window nothing could be seen; no building lights, no cars, nothing on the ground; even the wing tip lights were merely a soft glow some immeasurable distance away, obscured by a dense fog. Inside the cabin, 258 souls grew anxious; 13 hours in a plane at high altitude is mentally and physically debilitating.

An instant later, the 747's engines roared and a deep, powerful thrust sank me back into my chair. The pilot fought for altitude in what was an aborted landing in Beijing. For the next two hours we circled at 18,000 feet: no information, no explanation, fully unnerving. 30 minutes later, the passengers were informed that the plane could not land in Beijing: there was no visibility and we were proceeding to Hohhot. The pilot announced we would be landing in an hour; the Chinese passengers erupted in laughter.

The flight map on the screen in front of me provided no information at all on Hohhot (pronounced Who-heh-how-teh with heavy emphasis on the H consonants) other than its location…which was a long way away from Beijing. Looking at the map, I surmised it was doubtful I would be able to get car service to deliver me to my hotel in the Capital anytime that evening. We landed at Hohhot airport at about 6pm and the plane pulled up to the terminal, there was an announcement which got those eager passengers who had already begin to stand up and sort out their carry-on luggage to sit back down. I looked out my window and could see four other jumbo jets: Cathy, Asiana, Emirates, Singapore…all with their cabin lights on and silhouettes of passengers in their seats.

At 9pm, flight 137's passengers began to get restless. The plane's food had run out, the water supply was exhausted and of course, the toilet's function ceased. The flight attendants, who had been given no information on our circumstances, were frustrated with the constant questions by irate passengers. It was becoming evident that they were also victims of a wholly unprepared civil aviation authority. We were all stuck…at the mercy of some bureaucratic machine that wasn't prepared to offer us any information much less the services we required.

The next morning at 2am local time, 8 hours after landing in Hohhot and our 21st hour in the plane since leaving New York, a posse of angry passengers formed and began to give the flight attendants ultimatums. There was an attempt to open one of the cabin doors but when it was pointed out that there was no gangway and a leg-breaking 25 foot drop, they abandoned the effort. Other passengers were forming raiding parties and rummaging through the largely vacant first class cabins, collecting food, canned water and blankets. All order had now been abandoned and chaos was now upon us.

It was soon afterwards that we learned that the pilots had long ago left the plane to sleep in the terminal and with the growing anarchy, the flight attendants had lost their motivation to keep order. At 3am we were informed that ground crew had prepared for our disembarkation but it wasn't until 4am that we finally were led off the plane. In the terminal, which was dark except for some emergency lights we were greeted by a young lady who, dressed in full formal Mongolian dress, smiled with the reddest lipstick known to man and said repeatedly to the passengers as we filed off the plane: "Welcome to Hohhot, home of glorious Mongu peoples!" We were too numb to respond. Like sheep, they filed us into buses for some unknown destination.

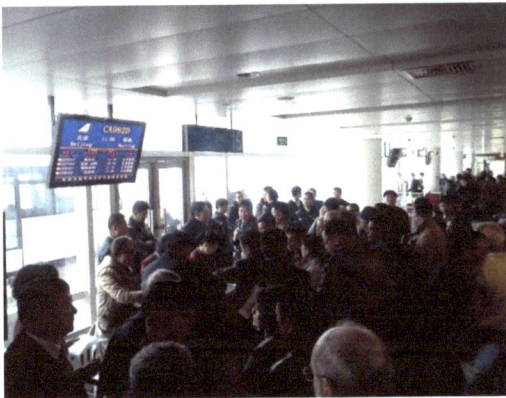

Figure 20 Stranded passengers fight for limited seats on a flight out of Hohhot

After two hours on the bus and two failed attempts to check into other hotels (the bus had taken us to the wrong hotel), all three buses arrived at a third and final hotel. During check-in, the hotel's concierge attempted to double bunk some passengers, myself and others resisted this forced camaraderie. I was finally processed and fell into my bed at 7am…26 hours after I left New York. As a parting word, before we began to head towards our rooms, our "administrator" who had been assigned to us by Air

China, told us to be prepared to leave the hotel at 9am to return to the airport for our trip back to Beijing. We ignored her.

But I did wake up at 9am and hurried myself to get ready, went downstairs and checked out. There were a few people in the lobby eating the stale rolls that had been placed next to a container of luke-warm tea. Of course, there was no sign of an impending departure and our China Air administrator was nowhere to be found. So I wandered outside into a dry, biting cold and out onto the street hoping I might find something fresher to eat and possibly a cup of coffee.

Hohhot has nothing of the sort…or at least the part of town I found myself in was not going to satisfy me. My quarter of Hohhot was clearly a working class neighborhood, wide industry-size boulevards with nothing but local noodle shops on either side. In front of most shops, either on the sidewalk or in the street were large fires heating big pots of some food; men and women wrapped tightly in dark blue quilted coats and furry hats huddled around the fires using chopsticks to eat a slurpy mixture from their bowls. I looked down the street at the succession of open fires and it felt like a scene from the movie _Mad Max_, anarchistic and Armageddon like. I approached a man who seemed in charge of the first noodle shop as I walked down the boulevard.

In my best Mandarin I asked, "Do you have coffee?

He turned and looked at me, a little surprised to see a Lao-Wai in his shop.

With a quick snap of his head his gravelly voice scraped "Mei You"

I expected this...I turned and walked back the other way. After about two miles I still could not find that cup of coffee. But in my brief journey I did see enough of Hohhot which convinced me that, although the city is the political seat of Inner Mongolia, this is a very small place as Chinese cities go. There is also very little here...a monument to former Buddha glory and one to the dairy industry which dominates the local business...but not much else. It is a grey, nearly characterless city....emphasis on grey and characterless. The people who worked at the hotel and those I saw along the street personified the grey and characterless theme... they looked as if they were serving a dreaded life sentence in some hard labor camp. Perhaps the summer is nicer, but I'm not interested in finding out.

It wasn't until 2pm in the afternoon that we were pushed into a bus that took us back to the airport. Once there we had to fight our way through a crowd of nearly 4,000 stranded passengers. Security had been reduced to walking past a gauntlet of local police who eyed-balled you head to toe. Once at the gate, fights broke out among exasperated passengers trying to get in line. As we were herded into the plane at 4pm, the young lady with the red lipstick who had greeted us when we landed was back again. She smiled, gesturing like she was hugging all. In an overly grateful voice, she beseeched us: "Thank you for visiting glorious Mongu peoples... please come again!" Her unbridled enthusiasm further exhausted me. Most passengers ignored her but I forced a simile and thought to myself, knowing Hohhot as I do, it has been a long time since the glory days of Altan Khan and his father Kublai.

As the plane taxied along the tarmac, the sun came out. I was sitting in a window seat leaning against the side of the plane feeling numb from my 35 hour journey. The plane came to a full stop at the head of the runway as if to catch its breath for the final 2 hour leg of this tiresome journey. The pilot released the brakes and gunned the engines and the plane lumbered down the runway slowly gaining speed. I yawned and we lifted into the air. As we passed over the depressingly grey city of Hohhot, I could make out the familiar fires lit in the streets to cook food; the City's boundaries were sharp – housing, streets, cars all came to a sudden end and fields began. As the 747 gained altitude, it banked hard back to the east and for the first time I could see the countryside of Hohhot...the sun was low and behind us now illuminating the ground below in a silvery green which revealed beautiful rolling hills with cattle grazing as far as the eye could see. It reminded me of Iowa or perhaps Nebraska.

I had long ago learned it was futile to become excited about such ordeals. In China, these trials are a fact of life and all the outrage, hostility and indignation one develops is wasted energy. It's best to save the effort and search for positive opportunities within the present misery that is involuntarily thrust upon you. At this point, the prospect of rest was reward enough for my patience. I began to fall asleep thinking...Hohhot...home of glorious Mongu peoples...grey cement on the inside, green hills on the outside.

Charlie Chan and The Case of
The Missing Chinese Geriatrician
顶尖神探解开中国养老护理缺口之谜

同 志 们 好! Before I begin our investigation into this health care whodunit, a couple housekeeping items: First, I have created a mirror site www.chinaseniorliving.org as the Chinese government blocks my host, Wordpress, and therefore my formal CSL site www.chinaseniorliving.com is unavailable to my colleagues, clients and constituents in China. Many Mainlanders have asked for access to my essay so I decided to create a site accessible to them. The format is a little different but the content is identical. Second, the inspiration for this essay is twofold: on one hand is my interest in wanting to write a follow-up to my previous essay *Farewell my migrant health care worker* but haven't gotten around to it. In some way, this piece is a good echo as I address the general industry wide human resource issue albeit from a different perspective. On the other hand, I want to promote real answers for actual industry problems and not just ask rhetorical questions. Well, in due form, here is a solution to one of the big challenges we face....put your gumshoes on....***THE GAME IS AFOOT!*** [31]

I sat down with the venerable Detective Charlie Chan on the piers of Xiamen last week to discuss a mystery that has been frustrating the senior living industry in China of late, namely the dearth of adequately trained geriatric staff. Lucky to have such a moment with the brilliant detective, I wasted no time, "Detective, may I ask that you impart some of your investigatory powers to my quandary?"

---

31 This phrase was actually Sherlock Holmes and not Charlie Chan. It sounded good when I wrote it.

Charlie Chan, sitting across from me, supremely confident in his white linen suit and Panama straw hat, smiles and responds, "Grateful to assist any way, Ke Zong."

I nod in appreciative supplication as Chan addresses me respectfully as Chairman Cole. I begin, "Imagine, if you will Detective, a human resources paradise; a separate reality, a parallel universe, linguistically and culturally identical to China yet with a social welfare system advanced by, say, 25 years. Such a Shangri-La might offer "crystal ball" possibilities, a peek into the future if you will; experienced geriatric nurses, a proven and culturally acceptable business model for senior living enterprises to mention just a few, no? We in the senior living business here in China are in dire need of such a vision."

Detective Chan considers my statement carefully and ponders my dilemma. Stroking his short dark beard, he cocks his head slightly and gazes out from the shores of Fujian Province and over the 180 kilometer-wide Formosa Strait as a salty, sub-tropical air rushes over the pier. Charlie Chan, eyes focused on the horizon, responds cryptically as if speaking to the breeze, "Humble to suggest..... foolish to seek fortune when real treasure hiding under nose......"

After a brief moment, Chan slowly turns his head. His almond shaped eyes penetrate; he stares at me silently. I am suddenly aware of the gravity of his proposition, he has given me a clue and it has implications.....

Briefly....Charlie Chan

Early last century a wholly adorable detective persona was created by Earl Derr Biggers called Charlie Chan. He was loosely based on Honolulu detective Chang Apana; Biggers conceived of the benevolent and heroic Chan as an alternative to early 20th century Yellow Peril stereotypes, such as villains like Fu Manchu so prevalent at the time. Chan first appeared in Biggers' novels, but went on to be featured in a number of media including, believe it or not, comic books. Nearly four dozen films (47 to be

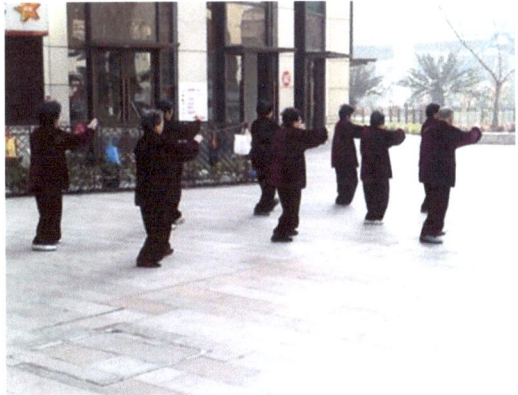

Figure 21 Early morning Tai-chi session for Shanghai elderly

exact) featuring Charlie Chan have been made, beginning in 1926. If you have seen any of the Chan pictures, he immediately reminds one of the more modern private eye incarnations such as the equally endearing and humble, yet mercilessly relentless, Detective Columbo; polite, inquisitive and always vexing to the guilty. Nearly as legendary as his finely honed detective skills was Charlie Chan's ability to pepper his dialogue with aphorisms delightfully appropriate to the moment. Whether he was tangled up in a dangerous situation or enjoying a quiet interlude with one of his many children, Mr. Chan always had a timely truth poised on the tip of his trenchant tongue.

The character was at first portrayed by Asian actors, and the films (3 of them) met with little success. In 1931, the Fox Film Corporation cast Swedish actor Warner Oland (of Shanghai Express fame and Essay Post #6…) as Chan in *Charlie Chan Carries On*; the film was a box office blockbuster, and Fox went on to produce 15 more Chan films with Oland in the title role. After Oland's death, American actor Sidney Toler was cast as Chan; Toler made 22

Chan films, first for Fox and then for Monogram Studios. After Toler's death, six more films were made starring Roland Winters.

The crime scene

A few weeks ago, eager to pursue Chan's hint that a possible solution involved a place on the horizon, I flew from Beijing south and across that 180 kilometer-wide, cerulean Formosa Strait to visit the tiny island of Taiwan, on an investigation to a place I lived for nearly 5 years in the 1970's. Early one morning I boarded Air China flight 185, as if I had a search warrant in hand armed with the fervor of CPC police in pursuit of political dissidents.

I was once told that if you really want to know a city in which you are a visitor, wake up early and walk. Watching how a city gets out of bed and starts its day reveals its heart and soul. So, on my first morning back in Taipei, in due fashion, I woke up at 5:30am and began to walk around....up and down Zhongshan North Boulevard, under ribbons of dizzy, soaring freeway overpasses.... as the sanitation trucks, operated by men and women laughing at each other's jokes, wrestled with foul smelling bags of rotten food. The street sweepers whistled while shop owners washed and scrubbed their sidewalks clean of the night's grit. This may seem a little Disney-like but in large part it is true, Taipei has grown up; it is a pleasant place at that hour in the morning. But now, at 6:30am after the City's first cup of jasmine tea, this day dream ends and things do of course change. Despite the charm of an early Taipei morning, its days are oppressively hot; the humidity dominates, the pollution asphyxiates and the congestion incarcerates.

In the early 1970's Taiwan struggled; citizens had few freedoms, frequently censored media, and a burgeoning manufacturing center of goods deemed cheap knockoffs by most. But time and prosperity cure many things and today the island stands in stark contrast to what it was back then. Contemporary Taiwan is a thoroughly modern, first world economy and an Asian center for technological innovation. Its citizens enjoy rich civil rights (wait...littering, spitting and other objectionable, antisocial behavior has been outlawed and infractions are punished with near Singaporean-like severity. The result is, however, notably clean streets and subways) and, comparatively speaking, Taiwanese have a comfortable standard of living. The island has a population of just about 23 million, roughly the size of Beijing; Taiwan's over-65 demographic is 2.5 million with an average life expectancy of nearly 80 years. Sure, Taiwan is little, but remember what Chan says about packaging:

"Humbly suggest not to judge wine by bottle"
Charlie Chan's Greatest Case

Thirty five years ago, Taiwan was governed by the authoritative and strong armed Kuomintang, Chiang Kai-shek's Nationalist Party which fled from mainland China in 1949 having essentially lost its battle against Mao's communist party. Today, the island is a multi-party democracy with an opposition candidate having won the presidential election for the first time on March 18, 2000. The peaceful transfer of power from the Kuomintang to the Democratic Progressive Party validated Taiwan's democratic political system. To my mind, Taiwan's social and political success is evidence of what an emerging pluralistic democracy can achieve; witness: the disproportionately large effect on the world economy which the small Chinese population of Taiwan has had. And while the United States can rightfully take some credit for providing a safe haven for such prosperity to flourish, the Taiwanese were/are driven and continue to be eager for even greater successes.

The forensic evidence

All good mysteries are founded and solved on the discovery and development of clues. Clues are, of course, developed based on a preponderance of evidence, intuition for the nature of the crime and an insight into the motivation of the perpetrator. Well, we don't really have a crime here nor do we have a culprit or I should say, without proof as of yet, the alleged guilty party. But since those of you who are reading this have likely read my previous essays, you appreciate the liberties I take with story lines.

My clues here are based on the evidence I found at the CCRC's I visited in Taiwan and the interrogation (again, my liberties) of a unique industry professional. The questioning of my witness follows the presentation of the evidence. At the end of the story I set forth my final argument and hope you are as convinced as I.

Clue #1: My first investigation turned up Chang Gung Health and

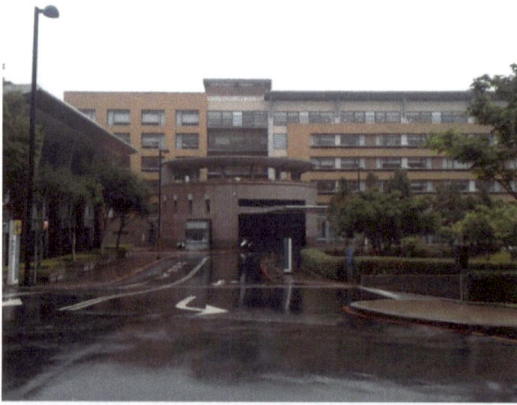

Figure 22 Chang Gung facility, Taoyuan Taiwan

Culture Village, a large CCRC 30 minutes from downtown Taipei and 15 minutes to the (new) airport, Chiang Kai-Shek International airport, in Taoyuan. Chang Gung is the brain child of one of Taiwan's wealthiest and most philanthropic minded entrepreneurs, Mr. Yung-Ching Wang. In its present configuration the facility, built in 2005, is comprised of 700 independent and assisted living units and a 250 unit nursing facility. The facility is about 75% occupied. I believe the reason for the low occupancy is that the primary access road has been under construction for about a year and a half; it is an unpleasant journey and must kill the sales process before it even begins. The entire land area at Chang Gung will ultimately be built out with another 15 buildings with a total of 3,000 senior living units; to be sure, an impressive and large facility.

Chang Gung is owned by the Chang Gung system of hospitals and like the hospitals it is a private facility. Naturally, the facility has a direct agreement with the Chang Gung hospital (located 3 kilometers from the CCRC) to provide preferential, emergency health care to the residents of the CCRC and there are a number of ambulances to quickly shuttle residents if need be.

By Taiwan standards, Chang Gung is affordable. The facility leases rooms based on annual rental. There are two unit sizes, a 22 ping[32] unit and a 14 ping unit. These units rent for NT26,000[33] per month and NT18,000 per month with a surcharge of NT5,000 per month for an additional person. In order to rent a unit, a deposit of 12 months is required. A package deal is available which includes meals and activities (an extra NT4,500). Chang Gung has an assisted living program which essentially includes 2 hours of social worker or nursing attention on a daily basis. This program costs NT10,000 per month.

What strikes me as important about Chang Gung isn't their facility at all but the quality of their staff. Each nurse and every social worker hold university degrees in their fields and special certificates for geriatric care. These geriatric care certificates are not bestowed

---

32 The unit of measurement that a ping represents is equal to about 3.3 square meters. These units would therefore be roughly equal to 650 sq. ft and 415 sq. ft., respectively.

33 The conversion rate of NT to USD is about 29:1.

as a result of a quick 20 hours of classroom work but require no less than 8 months of both classroom study and clinical experience. Further, Chang Gung's nurses are all members of a nurse union or other labor union which requires maintenance of professional standards

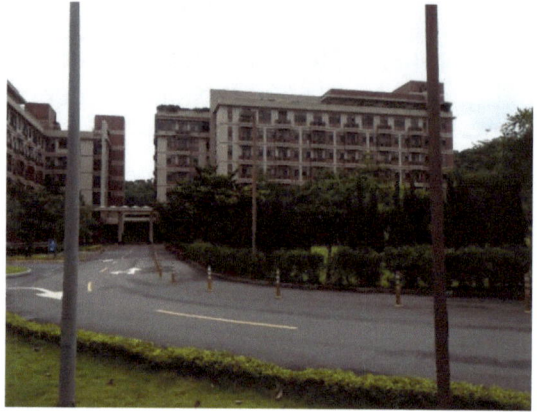

Figure 23 Suan Lien facility, Taipei

among their rank and file. These unions also lobby Taiwan's legislature to advance the status and financial security of nursing in Taiwan. If nothing else evidence of unionization is an undeniable clue to the fact that nursing is deemed an important job and one that has growing status in Taiwan society.

Clue #2: Later that morning I got back into the mini-bus, generously provided by Bruce Liu of 55 Tone, and headed north to the seaside community of Sinchi, about an hour from Taipei. We arrived at Suan Lien Elder Home: a 250 room CCRC owned and administered by the Presbyterian Church of Taiwan (this CCRC is a public facility and not exclusively for those of the Presbyterian faith). For a CCRC it is small, but the hardware at Suan Lien, which was built in 2000, is well maintained. I would grade the buildings and interior highly.

Again, the impressive thing here isn't the facility although like Chang Gung it is attractive, many rooms have ocean views. Suan Lien's pricing is not much different from Chang Gung; the differences amount to a slightly higher initial deposit and a special medical deposit for dementia patients (the term memory care has not yet come to Asia). The dementia care wing at Suan Lien is the best I have seen to date in Asia (ex. Japan) and is based on what they refer to as "unit care". The Suan Lien is 100% full and it has a waiting list of over 1,000 people. It is regarded as one of the best retirement homes on Taiwan. Why? Simple, the quality of the staff and the support of an organization trusted by the Taiwanese to deliver care of the highest caliber. Even the Taiwan government has taken notice; it provides Suan Lien with a subsidy of over NT5 million to augment their care program. Here is the grand finale; Suan Lien's budget has a dedicated line item to allocate 10% of their beds to low income persons[34]. Consider the evidence here: the presence of faith-based senior living organizations can be a sign of a higher commitment to care and can be an indication of superior care quality. But to add to this government financial support and self-imposed low income beds....I find this to be a subtle but strong clue of an advanced industry. As Chan would say:

"Little things tell big story" _Charlie Chan in London_

Clue #3: I lingered at Suan Lien a bit too long and my host, Bruce Liu, had to shuffle my team and me back into our transport and rush us to our last stop of the day: Jen Shi Citizens Rest Home. Jen Shi is located back near Taipei in a suburb called Dam Shui. This facility, with only 122 beds, is the smallest I saw while in Taipei and the oldest, having been built in 1960. The original facility was torn down in 2002 and rebuilt into its current configuration. The facility operates today at 92% occupancy.

Again, pricing at Jen Shi is not meaningfully different and I found the staff of equal if not better quality than both Chang Gung and

---

34 I asked if the government financial support required the allocation of low income beds and they said no. The allocation of low income beds is self-imposed by the Church.

Suan Lien. What struck me about Jen Shi was the facility manager, Chen Wei-Ping. Wei Ping is a woman, I estimate in her early forties, and has been the manager of Jen Shi for 10 years. Always smiling, she has a friendly but commanding personality and highly

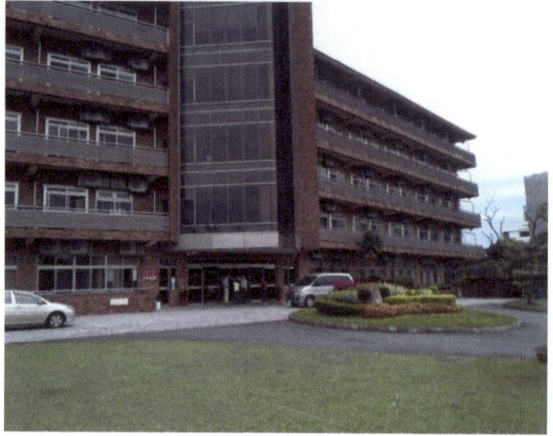

Figure 24 Jen Shi Rest Home, Taipei

sure of herself. As we toured the facility, she clearly has the admiration of her staff as they all paid respectful notice to her in passing. Moreover, each resident we met broke into open conversation with her almost as if they were finishing a chat started just a few minutes before I arrived. Wei Ping is clearly engaged with her facility in a manner I have not seen yet in Asia; she is fully immersed with her residents and staff. She lives and breathes her responsibility at Jen Shi.

While we were walking the halls I had the chance to ask her about care standards. She reported that Taiwan's Ministry of the Interior created the Bureau of Social Welfare nearly 8 years ago. This Bureau is charged with the inspection and enforcement of many different social welfare functions in Taiwan, including retirement homes. Every 3rd year, they do a comprehensive inspection of every senior living facility in Taiwan, its care program, staff credentials and resident interviews. Ah, my last clue: State enforcement and management of standards in any business is irrefutable evidence of an advanced or at least developing industry.

The smoking gun

Late on my second day in Taipei, I interrogated my primary witness, Dr. Shyh-Dye Lee, M.D., a valuable informant: he is the founder of Taiwan's Graduate Institute of Long Term Care, a professor at the National Taipei University of Nursing and Health Sciences and the current Chairman of the LTC Association, founded in 1994.

Professor Lee came to the meeting in what I came to learn during the course of our chat is his typically serious demeanor; I was lucky to meet with the Professor. He is a solemn person and discusses the status of senior living in Taiwan in a humorless manner as if preaching to the unfaithful; like Chen Wei Ping, Professor Lee is driven...dedicated to a selfless vocation of improving the status and quality of senior care to the Taiwanese elderly; he is a jewel in the crown for Taiwan's aged care industry. During the course of my examination, I was struck by his mastery of aged health care; using vocabulary such as mobility indices, tertiary preventive care programs, and non-pharmacological interventions for dementia; the Professor is unimpressed with fancy facilities and high-end amenities, he is simply, wholly absorbed with the advancement of care and caring.

Professor Lee struggles with trying to help Taiwan evolve with what the West experienced in the 1990's namely, the "Culture Change Movement". His single most important mission? Attempting to advance Taiwan's understanding and practice of gerontology from a medical model of care to a philosophy of wellness....a noble calling, indeed.

My time with Professor Lee was invaluable and proved to me that he has no Mainland counterpart. He has been to China and laments the "real estate cum service model" trap to which many elderly are falling prey. When asked to point out aged care differences between Taiwan and China, he holds forth with encyclopedic knowledge of Taiwan's geriatric care industry regulations such as *Senior Citizens Welfare Living Allowance Provisional Act*[35], which provided all those over the age of 65 with additional state funds to be used for aged care if required. Legislation such as this clearly sets Taiwan above and beyond China's present status and is a model that should be studied. I am immediately reminded again of Chan's wisdom when thinking of Professor Lee's functional lack of a peer in China:

"Man who improve house before building foundation, apt to run into very much trouble" ***The Feathered Serpent***

I don't want to overstate my case here. In all reality there may be an aged care specialist or two in China whose breadth of experience, understanding and drive is a good match with the Professor's; after all, I have not undertaken a census of all geriatric care professionals in China. However, I doubt it, and even if there are, I am willing to wager that Professor Lee is certainly not unique in Taiwan; there are plenty of experienced clinical geriatricians on the island all of whom speak Mandarin, are ethnic Chinese and thus represent a precious pool of human resources. It takes time to build an arsenal of geriatric care professionals. It's a tough job with a lousy reputation. Think about it…they care for frail, vulnerable humans, they feed them, wash them…they are in close, intimate contact with them at all times. In a sense and at some length, they develop deep relationships with their patients. And then, the patient dies and the nurse has to do it all over again the next day. The burnout rate is heavy.

---

35 Promulgated by President Order Hua-Tsung (1)-Yi-Tzu No.09100100580 on May 22, 2002

Mystery solved, case closed!

In sum, the strategic advantages offered by Taiwanese skilled labor have been wholly overlooked by senior living companies looking to gain a foothold in the China market to date. I have 3 reasons to believe that Taiwan serves as a likely source, if not the leading provider, of senior living, nursing and LTC human resources (not to mention a model for building and care standards) for the near future:

1) Taiwan is nearly identical linguistically to mainland China; at most there is a slight accent that separates them,
2) Taiwan and China are culturally and ethnically very similar to each other, and
3) In a social welfare and a public health context, Taiwan is no less than 25 years ahead of China.

I don't mean to suggest that Taiwanese skilled labor offers a panacea for China's senior living industry or that the industry's structure is a jig for China's; in fact, my point is far from this notion. To wit, the Chinese love affair with western brands will certainly preclude this from ever taking place, however misplaced this infatuation may be. My point is better understood through another of Detective Chan's aphorisms:

"Good tools shorten labor" ***Charlie Chan at the Circus***

What the Taiwanese offer is simply a "plug and play" solution to certain temporary management /training roles for a Mainland CCRC or other geriatric service facility. Taiwanese geriatric nurses have the care skills, the language ability and their culture is a match; there are no cross-eyed stares, instead, understanding is seamless and without the problematic filter of interpretation. Now, the concept of the mainland using Taiwanese labor to improve their knowledge base is not a new phenomenon, in fact there are thousands of Taiwanese working in China; after all the pay is good and they have an edge.

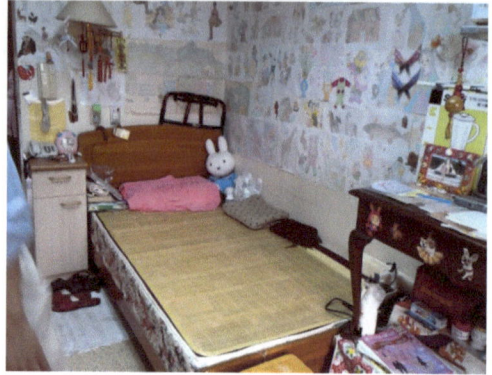

Figure 25 Resident's well decorated room at Jen Shi, Taipei

There are shortcomings however. Namely, this relationship doesn't last long; once the Chinese master the Taiwanese's skills, the liaison is often over as the imported labor is usually significantly more expensive. Also, there are some day to day sensitivities that need to be addressed with hands on management and understanding. These differences, borne out of the complex political relationship between Taiwan and China, should be viewed and treated like diversities and then won't prove fatal; think of these generally as the rivalry that occurs between siblings; one bigger and stronger the other smaller but smarter.

"If strength were all, tiger would not fear scorpion"
Charlie Chan's Secret

In my the previous essay, *All aboard!....this the China CCRC Express*, I set forth the "FIRE!.... Aim....Ready.....approach to geriatric care development in China. There are those in the China senior living industry today, the true players that live and work there, who are setting plans to construct training centers and proceeding along an "organic" method of building experienced teams of geriatric technicians. Ultimately, I am agnostic about this. On one hand I see the value of a home grown bench, if you will. On the other, I see it as an opportunity for endless frustration as such a valuable resource will undoubtedly be cherry picked mercilessly by the competition. At least temporarily, I tend to favor importing skilled labor over the expense of building a training facility and program. There will come a time for building training centers, I have no doubt, but in the meantime I will take my cue from Chan:

"Ideas planted too soon, often like seeds on winter ground – quickly die" ***The Sky Dragon***

Not only am I the detective here but I am also judge, jury and executioner, after all this is my essay. So in closing, I want to address yet another often suggested solution for staffing which I have seen attempted a couple of times. Namely, this is the use of translators to interpret between a western company's clinical experts, their managerial staff and local employees. Now, if we were talking about an assembly line production of widgets on a fast moving conveyor belt….the "inserting A into B and wrap with C"…type of job, and then I might wholly support the translator method of proceeding.

But the business isn't a production line, Gerontology and Geriatrics are the "fine medical arts". We are talking about caring for frail, infirm elderly Chinese persons who were born before the revolution and are likely slightly unmoored by the notion of living in a facility not to mention their apprehension with modern Chinese society in general. Now then, introduce into this mix John Q. Manager who has been in China for 6 months, standing next to his translator who is hastily trying to communicate Western aged care concepts, predicated on a Western government regulated delivery system of care, to a group of nurses educated in the Chinese health care system. While the two parties argue and misunderstand one another, the patient wanes.

I don't see this as a very practical solution. And while this doesn't preclude Western companies from participating in the China senior living industry, it does mean their approach must be nothing less than Chinese and not one predicated on what is done in Omaha, Nebraska or a one formulated from a Western framework.

Ah, so….the solution to the Case the missing Chinese geriatrician is a bit of a trick question…they aren't really missing today, they are just all in Taiwan.

Case closed.

I hadn't been back in Beijing for a day when I happened upon Detective Chan while out and about in the Guo Mao. Eager to report on my trip, I intercepted Chan as he walked towards the CCTV tower.

"Detective Chan!" I called out, "I've just returned from Taiwan I found some extraordinary information!"

"Ah, Ke Zong, grateful for surprise encounter!" Chan chirped as he shook my hand. The Detective leaned into me slightly and whispered, "Old police slogan: unusual thing always good clue."

I smiled warmly and responded with a wink. "Elementary my dear Mr. Chan[36], Old police slogan is true. I think you helped me solve an important mystery!"

"Difficult problem have many solution, Ke Zong." Chan counseled waving his index finger back and forth.

---

36 Op. cit footnote #31 !

"Yes, I know, Detective. And this mystery likely has a few but you also once told me "All solutions to same problem not created equal."

The Detective praised, "You learn fast, Ke Zong. It is good to see you back in Beijing!"

"Thank you Chan, It is good to see you again as well.....I have been meaning to ask your thoughts on another matter...regarding the operating model...."

Chan, sensing another mystery being placed at his feet, smiles as he turns to cross the street and cuts me off mid-sentence, "Always pleasant journey which ends among old friends, Ke Zong....." Chan's voice trailed off as he made his way into the cross walk.

Frantic to keep his attention, I interject, "But.....Detective, it won't take but a min...."

But the sleuth is too swift and slides out into the street. Halfway to the other side Chan turns, lifts his straw hat and nods at me, "Must let student solve other mystery by self....humble Detective have important appointment with gerontologist" Chan reaches the curb as the lights change and squadrons of motorbikes charge loudly into the intersection partially obscuring him. I catch a fleeting glimpse of the Detective's white linen suit as he recedes into the swarm of noonday foot traffic....watching as his hat appears once, bounces between heads, then disappearing into the crowd.

Intermission: Shanghai Nuptials on the ¼ Mile
中场片段: 老上海赛马厅之现代相亲角

One morning in late 1934, a crowd of foreign men, British, Americans and Germans, all dressed in morning suits and fine, black silk top hats gathered in front of the newly built Shanghai Race Club[37]. In was mid-September and the heat of day was already overbearing not to mention the wilting Huangpu River humidity. As the clock in

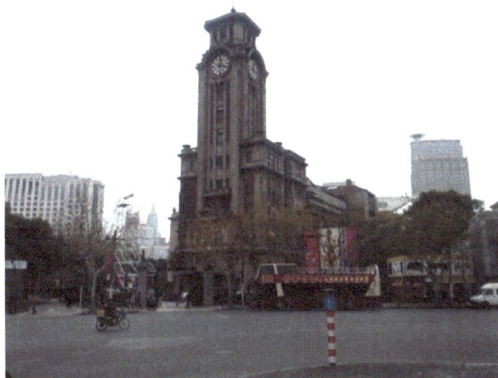

Figure 26 Clubhouse for the Shanghai Race Track built 1934

the building's tower struck 10am, A.W. Burkill, O.B.E. the Chairman of the race course flanked by his stewards stepped out from under the canopy and announced the commencement of the 72nd autumn race season and that fall's Shaforce Challenge Cup. While Burkill droned on and on about race protocol, the ladies of members, arm-in-arm and dressed in fine Irish linen gowns, each of whom carried a bright white parasol, strolled in front of the largest race track grandstand in Asia.

This tradition, already nearly a century old, was to end shortly as the political situation in China galloped towards full war. In 1937, Japanese would occupy all non-international portions of Shanghai and by 1941 even those "safe areas" were to capitulate to the Imperial army. As expected in this same year, along with the ceding of what remained of Shanghai to Japan, the Club closed. Its stout

---

37 The Shanghai Race Club was formally declared an independent club in 1862. Architects for the club house on Xizang Road were Spence, Robinson & Partners, Contractor was AH Hong &Co. The civil engineering firm was C. Luthy & Co.

granite walls built to withstand a century or more of continuous equestrian pleasures, festive derbies and exhilarating races, was became a stable for storing the Communist Party's munitions. A few years later in 1949, after the conclusion of the Chinese civil war, gambling and horse racing were found to be anathema to the doctrines of Communism. The Shanghai Race Club was outlawed and the premises were seized in the name of the people. It is unclear when but obviously sometime after 1949, the horse track was converted into People's Square; today it is a verdant park which attracts thousands of people each day who stroll along the outlines of the former horse track.

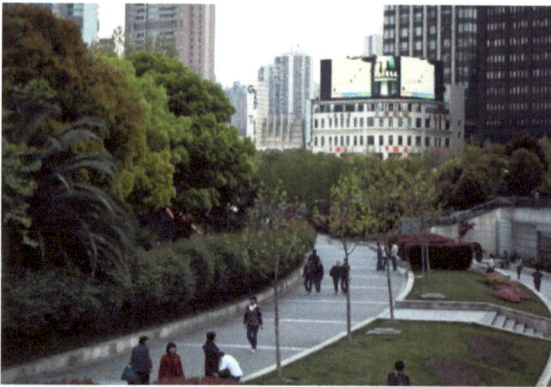

Figure 27 People's Square: the former horse track of the Shanghai Race Club (Wkpd)

On a recent weekend in Shanghai, I walked into People's Square seeking to mingle and enjoy a sunny September afternoon. As I passed from the east side of the square to the west, I found myself in a curious part of the park. Hundreds of elderly Chinese stood calling out to each other, beckoning as if at an auction; eagerly trying to attract attention to a placard which they guarded like some prized thoroughbred in a stable ready for stud. On each placard there was a picture, some were of a young man and others, a young woman. I stopped to read one particularly well decorated poster. Here is what it said:

"Seeking handsome young man from established professional family for our beautiful daughter. No visible

birthmarks, no handicaps. Must be between 25 and 35, earn over 500,000rmb per year salary. Must own apartment (without mortgage) of 150m2 inside 3rd ring road. Must give my daughter time deposit of 100,000RmB upon engagement, hand over monthly paycheck/yearly bonus and provide daily nanny care once daughter is pregnant. Must have western-style car of 200,000rmb minimum value...all credentials checked thoroughly. Serious applicants only"

Impressed with the outlandish demands listed, I turned my head from this placard and looked down the pathway in this section of the park...I could visibly make out what must have been 500 more such advertisements. This was a marriage market I surmised; proud Chinese parents busy scurrying

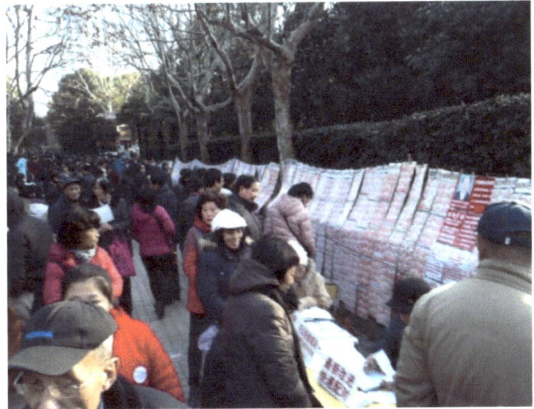

Figure 28 Marriage market People's Square, Shanghai

about making marriage deals on behalf of their children, selling the accomplishments of their adult child, arguing pedigree, bargaining for better terms, dismissing as baseless the perceived diminution of value caused by a unfortunate mole, etc., etc. And the adult children themselves? Absent of course...and likely disinterested.

Ah...I thought...the park has merely jumped from one sport to another...no longer a horse track but Shanghai's modern day marriage track. A lot of conclusions can be drawn from the activity every weekend on the west side of People's Square, many of which are misguided. Yet there is one truth that occurs to me every time

I pass by the Shanghai marriage market: Chinese parents are so thoroughly devoted to ensuring the success of their offspring that they spend their weekends searching for suitable wife or husband for their adult children.

I am only surprised that I am no longer surprised by what I encounter in Shanghai.

The China (senior living) Syndrome
中国养老供需综合征

"What makes you think they're looking for a scapegoat?" asks Jack Godell
"...Tradition..." snaps Ted Spindler in <u>The China Syndrome</u>

<u>The China Syndrome</u>, starring Jack Lemmon, Jane Fonda and Michael Douglas, was a gripping 1979 drama about the potential dangers of nuclear power. The term, China Syndrome, refers to a catastrophic accident, the fictional result of the meltdown of a nuclear reactor beginning with the loss of coolant fluid in the reactor and the partial or complete exposure of the fuel element assemblies. The core elements melt and burn through the containment vessel, the housing building and then notionally through the crust and body of the Earth until reaching the other side of the planet, which in the United States is popularly said to be China.

However, in reality, the physics of a China Syndrome is widely held to be unrealistic for a number of reasons, most notably, gravity. Yet, a large hole, hundreds of miles deep and thoroughly contaminated for thousands of years with deadly radiation is troublesome enough. In similar fashion, a China *senior living* Syndrome is my fanciful account of what I see as a potentially impaired market based on unrestrained, wildly speculative development of senior facilities without commensurate establishment of operating businesses much less proper strategic planning in advance of such schemes. Such a scenario would retard operational growth for quite some time. Although I call it a fanciful account, my staff and I have done a significant amount of research which I believe wholly supports the conclusions.

It is still early days for this industry and China is, after all, not the most transparent environment for data collection. However, development of presentations which attempt to resolve industry issues should not be binary, meaning a best efforts analysis or not....I mean, it is possible to make studied deductions based on market observations and offer them up for debate without access to reams of data. Insightful presentations can be done in a detailed manner and while they may not carry the weight of an academic, full market scan using tons of publically available, indisputable data; they are helpful if for nothing else than high quality debate.

On the second and last day of the Retirement Living World (IMAPAC) conference held in 2012, I was told that my presentation offered up data that no one had yet seen in China. Indeed, I firmly believe that is the following is the first attempt at a supply/demand evaluation of the China senior living market. Here is my hypothesis and what I said:

Hypothesis:

"Near term growth of supply in China senior living assets, particularly the high-end lifestyle product, may significantly outpace demand and if true, the resulting imbalance is likely to persist for the mid-term..."[38]

The fuel rods

The driver of China's nascent senior living industry is of course its demographics and much has been made of this phenomenon. Not that the demographics of China aren't unusual in their structure or amazing in their enormity, they are indeed; but I have found the attraction to the data and their use to be wholly without critical assessment. For example, everyone speaks about the 170 million Chinese seniors over the age of 65...and this is indeed the figure which has been reported by the various Chinese authorities and supported

---

38 Bromme H. Cole speech at IMAPAC conference Shanghai 2012

by the China Research Center on Ageing (CRCA). But this figure is a gross number and hasn't been vetted for those characteristics which might preclude one's use of a senior living facility, which characteristics are namely income and other cultural inclinations. In fact, as of today, no one has really attempted to qualitatively assign a size to what I call the China Senior Living cohort (CSL cohort). The question is: what is the population cohort that can be reliably measured/thought of as consisting of persons that have the requisite characteristics to consider a senior living facility?

Fact is, there are no indisputable figures that would lead one to an unquestionable calculation of the size of the CSL cohort. But I have done a bit of work in on this figure, such as a conjoint analysis of 550 elderly persons, estimates of the number of those older Chinese who earn over RmB250,000 per year and careful review of certain luxury retail sales from which inferences can be made about population size as well as other observations. Based on these analyses, I strongly believe the CSL cohort of Chinese seniors from whom senior living facilities will draw their residents is today approximately 10.2 million or roughly 6% of the total population of Chinese 65 and older (170 million). This CSL cohort will expand 12% over the next 4 years to approximately 11.4 million by 2016 based on standard population growth estimates provided by the CRCA.

The reactor

Over the past three years, I have traveled from Harbin to Sanya, from Shanghai to Chengdu in my search for and examination of senior living projects in China; my interest lies in their construction not only from a size, design and physical point of view but also in the development of their service and aged-care operations. The result from this exploration has been a database of projects replete with relevant information on their construction, operations, cost and occupancy among other critical industry data. To my knowledge, this data yields the only available metrics on the current supply of senior living in China.

At present, based on my personal observations, I know there to be approximately 25[39] (give or take a few) senior living projects in China. I define "senior living projects" as 1) a western style residential project, 2) built in the last 5 years, 3) specifically constructed and intended for adults over the age of 60, 4) age appropriate amenities for recreation and living support and, 5) offering any one or combination of the following living accommodations: independent living, assisted living and aged-care or skilled nursing capabilities. As a concrete example, this list would include such well known projects as Yue Cheng in Beijing, Yanda International Healthy City in Hebei province and Qinggang Elderly Nursing Center in Chongqing.

It should be well noted that I am not making any distinction between strata title projects, rental projects or any other unique operating characteristic such as a membership program. This analysis is a broad, industry wide compilation of projects which adhere to the 5 criteria set forth above. I readily admit that this is somewhat of an indiscriminate enquiry and as such may restrict the extent to which I can make accurate projections, but we have to start somewhere. Here are some further data on the present inventory and relevant supply conclusions:

1) Current supply has a present total bed count of 12,500 (average of 500 beds per project);
2) There is a total census (occupancy) in these projects of 4,250 yielding an industry wide occupancy of 35%;

---

39 An accurate number in June 2012. Today the figure is approximately 35.

3) Using the CSL cohort figure of 10.2 million, it would seem the current penetration rate is approximately .04% (only relevant when compared with western industry standards of 6%-7%).

Loss of coolant

Measuring future supply and demand is a wholly different matter and this exercise really relies entirely on my firm's presence in the market place and our care in noting all projects currently in planning (i.e., architectural drawings complete and ownership of land) or under construction. This is simply because there is no clearing house for such data presently in China; no one keeps track of these projects, collectively. So other than what we have gathered here, one would need to go out and spend 12 months counting projects, which is the next best alternative. Again, our data on these figures come directly from clients, discussions with prospective clients and visits to local planning commissions, government officials and the projects themselves.

Our data, with respect to future supply, is as follows:

1) There are 450 new projects currently under planning throughout China, of which I believe 75% (allowing for 25% attrition or cancelled projects) will be completed in 2-5 years;

2) If completed, these projects will produce a new supply of 168,750 new beds (500 bed average) yielding a total bed inventory of 181,250 beds.

The vastly more difficult aspect of this exercise is determining what future demand will be. We have long discussed this at my firm, consulted with CRCA colleagues and we broadly agree that no calculus exists today to estimate future senior living demand. So, after much deliberation, we decided to simply ask a different question, namely: What level of demand would be necessary to achieve two threshold scenarios: 1) an industry wide 75% occupancy (liminal profitability scenario) and, 2) an industry wide 40% occupancy (meltdown scenario) once all 168,750 new beds came online?

1) *Scenario 1*: Sufficient demand growth to 75% occupancy (industry wide) requires 32x increase in bed occupancy (linear calculation of 136,000 occupied beds from 4,250) – penetration rate of 1.2%; and,

2) *Scenario 2*: Growth in demand to 40% occupancy (industry wide) requires 17x increase in bed occupancy (again linear: 72,500 occupied beds from 4,250) and penetration rate of .64%.

Taken alone and without any additional context, these are staggering growth figures and I believe, superficially unachievable. However, there are mitigants and these scenarios as they strictly appear above are not likely to occur. Yet some industry fallout, and some is the operative word, is inevitable.

Moderation of chain reaction

Like that mythical hole through the core of the earth, it is entirely possible that a China *senior living* Syndrome will not occur. I have at least 4 reasons as to why (all likely and reassuring):

1) *Capital constraints may restrict supply* – every developer in China (unlisted) needs cash today and without it he is unlikely to pursue further real estate development;

2) *Lumpy, inefficient market* – This analysis is admittedly theoretical for a number of reasons but most importantly because it is based on: i) an industry without publically available data, ii) gross, industry wide averages and iii) a fair share analysis which doesn't strictly apply in nascent market place situations. It is however, and I stress, not entirely far-fetched;

3) *Developer attrition* – Neophyte China senior living developers may opt out due to i) eventual realization that senior living isn't really a property business, ii) exceedingly long dated ROI and iii) high degree of complications with having to build operator;

4) *The China axiom* – Like the early 1990's Nokia cell phone lesson where great debate was held on how many mobile phones should be produced for their first manufacturing run...it was decided that 50 million was sufficient; they learned 3 months later that demand was actually 250 million. In essence, never underestimate China; demand could meet the theoretical supply.

Resumption of controlled fission

Yet, it would be unrealistic to imagine that some degree of over-capacity is improbable for the industry in the near term. In fact, with present occupancy at 35% we are already there. But even in the next two years with intensified excess supply, given the nature of an embryonic industry, it will be wholly possible for astute, well prepared developers to "beat the market" and exceed industry averages in terms of occupancy; I have no doubt about this. But preparation and market insight will be the threshold imperatives for such out-performance. Going forward, reliance on one's previous experience, be it western or local, will be inadequate. And finally in this regard, Good News! As a consequence to however severe or mild the over-capacity might be, I project that by 2014 the China senior living landscape will be populated with "value add" opportunities or a new age in distressed investing where the winners are masters of both the real estate and operating sides of the business.

With this essay, I am clearly revising my thoughts on the China senior living market. It is not a negative revision at all; I am just fine tuning my outlook to accommodate near term choppy waters. In the long term, I remain very positive. I live, eat and sleep this business and see it evolving on a daily basis but no longer do I have the blind faith in the high-end market I once held: I am now agnostic and suggest a "hold" at best for this sub-sector. Further, the potential over supply and probable slow demand curve concerns me in the near term. I recommend going "long" on the mid to lower-mid range market or swap out to the sub-acute, skilled nursing sector; there's reliable data there and no catastrophic meltdown in sight.[40]

---

40 This analysis was performed and presented during the 2nd quarter of 2012. Since this time, additional data has become available. This new information has furthered our thoughts on the industry and matured our conclusions, even though many of the fundamentals remain the same.

Intermission: Dynastic Beijing
中场片段: 天子脚下的北京城

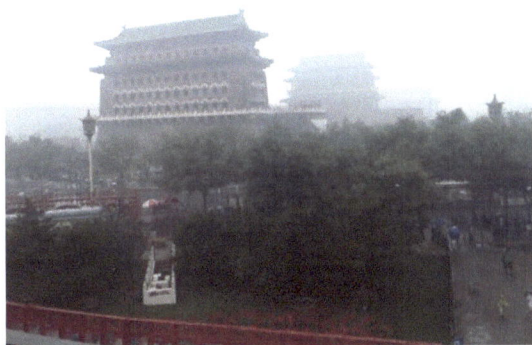

Figure 29 Qing and Ming Gates Qianmen, Beijing

Few cities in this world are more ostentatious than Beijing; she is pretentious and immodest, parading her authority grandly like some ornately adorned, Qing Dynasty Diyi[41]... its only real purpose: to instill envy and win admiration. Beijing is a rich city and nearly all Chinese influence, both corporate and political, are concentrated within her municipal territory. The city is China's center of gravity; Beijing rules like a harsh Dowager Empress intolerant of any dissent, commanding the distant corners of her empire with fiat...issuing decrees with the cold slap of her hand.

Despite a plethora of modern skyscrapers, Beijing is dominated architecturally by the Forbidden City, a wondrous place and the largest imperial compound in the world. It was built in the early 1400's and today consists of 980 surviving buildings arranged on 180 acres. The compound is quarantined within walls that are a towering 26 feet high and a 170 foot wide moat further separates it from the world. Despite its beauty, the purpose behind that alluring façade is clear: invulnerable fortress; the Forbidden City was designed to be impenetrable and consequently isolating. It is nevertheless enchanting and those who spent their lives impounded

41 Formal wear for a Princess or Empress.

behind its massive gates, sequestered deep within the labyrinthine complex of its structures, had little else to do but to dream up the most poetic names for these buildings. Among my favorite are the Palace of Tranquil Longevity, the Hall of Mental Cultivation and the Palace of Heavenly Purity.

The Forbidden City was home to 24 Ming and Qing Dynasty Emperors[42], their many concubines, large extended families, numerous court officials, useless retinues, hundreds of eunuchs, obsequious hangers-on, etc., etc. The histories of these Emperors are fairly complete; many were ruthless enriching themselves and expanding their territory at any cost, a few brought true peace and prosperity to China and of course, some were complete inbred dolts. A lot can be said of these two Dynasties but no one can label them uninteresting or colorless.

One of many...

Empress Dowager Cixi was born in Beijing on 29 November 1835 and died in the Forbidden City on 15 November 1908. She came from the Yehenara clan, a Manchurian family, and spoke both Mandarin and Manchu; she was a powerful, ruthless and charismatic woman. These traits along with a little luck enabled her to effectively rule the Qing Dynasty for 47 years. The dynasty fell three years after her death. Cixi spent most of her life ensconced within the walls of the Forbidden City in Beijing fomenting palace intrigue and designing imperial conspiracies.

Cixi came from humble beginnings, the daughter of a local Beijing low to mid-level official but ultimately lived a grand, self-important life. In her adolescence she was selected by the Xianfeng Emperor

---

42 The Ming were ethnic Chinese or Han people and the Qing were from Manchuria and known as Manchu people.

as an imperial concubine. In the concubine business, not unlike the Princess business in Europe during the Renaissance, if you produced a son you did well otherwise your role as a consort was at risk and the comfortable life you led within the Imperial Palace, tenuous. Indeed Cixi met the challenge and gave birth to Emperor Xianfeng's son, who became the Tongzhi Emperor upon his father's death in 1861. But Tongzhi was only 5 years old when he ascended the throne and therefore, Cixi, in order to protect her son's auspicious future and more importantly keep her place in the Forbidden City needed to oust a group of Regents appointed by the late Emperor. After all, there was no shortage of other concubines who wanted their sons to be Emperor. They would stop at nothing, not even infanticide, to realize this ambition. So given the mercurial nature of palace life, Cixi enlisted the help of her predecessor, Empress Dowager Ci'an, and did what she thought best. She allied herself with other shrewd Palace strategists, bargained for support and eventually consolidated control over the Qing Dynasty, executing a few of the Regents along the way

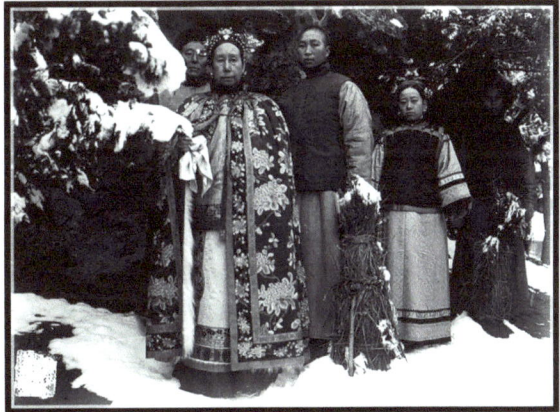

Figure 30 An elderly Empress Dowager Cixi with eunuchs (Wkpd)

in what has become known as the Xinyou Palace Coup. Cixi had proved herself a dominating force.

But by 1864 after having lost two Opium wars and suffering the expensive victory of the bloody Taiping Rebellion[43], China under the Qing, was unraveling. Cixi's answer: embark on a program of xenophobia: forbid Qing subjects to study abroad, consolidate forces, alienate the foreign embassies and refuse the construction of a railroad as it would disturb the Imperial Tombs. As she aged, her paranoia got the better of her.

Not surprisingly, Cixi was also an overbearing mother who engendered much suspicion among those surrounding Tongzhi. She was especially apprehensive about his young wife, the Empress Jiashun and mistrustful of her ambitions. As a remedy, Cixi decided to separate the two. This terminal error had the effect of driving Tongzhi to Beijing's brothels where he caught smallpox and died in 1875. Tongzhi passed without a male heir and so Cixi again needed to maneuver to protect her position and found what seemed like a suitable candidate in her nephew, Guangxu. Of course, Guangxu had a difficult rule as Cixi wouldn't cease her meddling. But he did manage to reign, albeit in name only, for over 30 years. Ultimately, his effectiveness as Emperor was diluted by the chaos resulting from Cixi's incessant interference, all of which contributed to the degeneration of the Qing Dynasty. These were the final days for the royal Manchus; China lost one battle after another...mainly to the Japanese and British. Sealing the Dynasty's fate as the 19th Century drew to a close, Cixi depleted the Qing's treasury on whimsies like the building of a grand Summer Place in a time when her armies sorely needed reinforcement and modernization.

---

43 The ruler of Taiping – current day Nanjing - Hong Xiuquan, believed he was the brother of Jesus Christ and in a fit of religious zeal, set about trying to over throw the Qing: it is estimated 25 million civilians died in this war and the famine that followed.

At the dawn of the 20th century, a new era was upon the Qing. Rebellions like the Boxer sprang up frequently as the Han and Manchu alike grew intolerant over increasing foreign control in China. In the days before her death, Cixi, afraid of the reforms Guangxu had enacted and unable to accept his continued rule without her surreptitious oversight, had him poisoned. A day after Guangxu's homicide, Cixi lay paralyzed on her deathbed. In a pitiful move, she installed a distant relative, Puyi, a toddler, as the 12th and final Qing Emperor. In the end, Cixi, a lowly born pretender to the Qing throne without so much as a drop of royal blood, died like she lived: a vain, paranoid and conceited Empress concerned only with protecting her position. Her final act: instructing the eunuchs to place a massive black pearl in her mouth after she died to protect her corpse from decomposing.

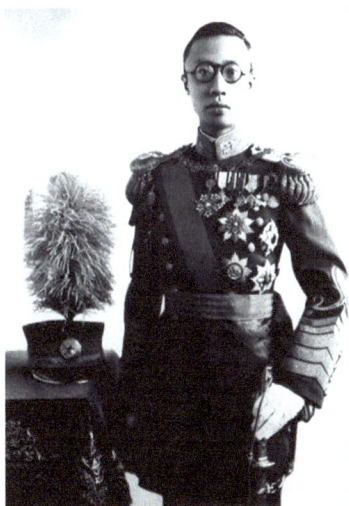

Figure 31 Puyi as Japanese in-stalled puppet-emperor of Manchuko (Wkpd)

And as for Puyi, he ascended the throne when he was 2 years old under the care of mischievous regents who knew the end of the Qing was near. They surrounded him like human vultures, looting what was left of the Palace's treasures while all the time pretending to be loyal court officials and doting advisors. The film *The Last Emperor* was insightful in telling his pathetic story; he was wholly unprepared to deal with the realities of a new China; the Qing disintegrated in 1912.

China, and the social changes wrought upon it by the neglectful Qing, had arrived at a new era which had no room for grand monarchs. Even if Puyi had been more adroit, it is unlikely that he would have been able to stem the tide of the inevitable revolution. The Qing treasury was empty and the desire among the Chinese for change was overwhelming. Yet even as an adult Puyi was hapless, he was incapable of reconciling himself with his reality as his interest lay in being a medal-festooned emperor relevant only to some bygone era. Ultimately, he was supported only by those interested in using him, be they the Regents of his childhood or the invading Imperial Army. And when the Japanese lost the war, Puyi's final charade ended; he was sentenced to rehabilitation by the Communists and died a sad, uneventful and largely forgotten death in 1968.

The story of the Qing's 268 year rule from within the walls of the Imperial Palace is a long, complicated tale full of intrigue, conspiracies and of course, betrayal. There were effective rulers as well as incompetent ones, a rise to the heights of absolute power and in the end, as most dynasties pass, an internal collapse: the result of ignorance bred from isolation. Ultimately, the Forbidden City, a beautiful garrison which so thoroughly protected the dynasties through the centuries, its massive parapets discouraging invaders and repelling assault after assault, could not safe-guard the Qing from themselves.

Like the Qing and the dynasties which preceded it, the current Chinese government is also complex and has its own share of internal plotting, brilliant heads of state and inept ones as well. But while the dynasties endured for centuries, the current government of China has been around for a mere 64 years...just a few years short of Cixi's age when she died.

What happens next in Dynastic Beijing is anyone's guess.

The Good Senior Living Operator
养 老 运 营 最 佳 舵 手

*"...five years is nothing in a man's life except
when he is very young and very old."*
*Pearl S. Buck, **The Good Earth***

The overarching theme in Pearl S. Buck's *The Good Earth* is the nourishing and regenerative power of the land; connections with the earth are associated with moral piety, good sense, respect for nature, and a strong work ethic, while alienation from the land is connected with decadence and corruption. In a similar fashion, filial piety is a central, almost universal theme within the context of traditional Chinese culture and its intra-familial relationships. Estrangement from this custom has led and will continue to lead to the unmooring of a generation and disaffection within Chinese families.

For those of you who might be expecting a posting with insight into the senior living market in China or yet more information on supply/demand forces may be disappointed with this piece; it hasn't much of either. I am taking a small essay-break and delving into a little creative writing. But even as I say that I must correct myself and admit that I am indeed writing about the industry, only from a different narrative. In fact, rather than calling this posting "The Good Senior Living Operator", I could, were I so inclined to dismiss my interest in China-themed film and literature, call it the "Anti-brand Senior Living Operator"; but that wouldn't be nearly half as fun, now would it? Yes, there is a sub-text to this story...a business proverb of sorts, and it is one that I have been exploring for some time. If you wish, read and find out more.

This is a wholly fictional story about a Chinese developer who at the pinnacle of his career and having made a towering fortune in developing real estate, experiences the wrenching and painful death of his father, Wang Xiaoping. Despite all his wealth, Wang Xi was frustrated that he could not provide his father more comfortable, focused care. This experience cascades into a catharsis for Wang Xi; from that point forward he dedicates his life to the altruistic endeavor of caring for the elderly and spends a good portion of his

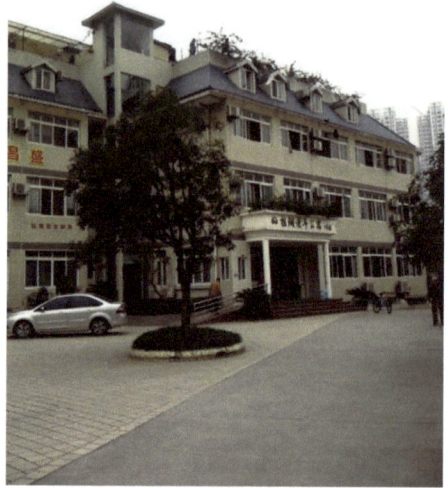

Figure 32 Guihou Senior Living facility, Chongqing

wealth on improving their lives and comforting them in their dotage. In his epic journey, Wang Xi comes to eschew the trappings of modern society and returns to fundamental Chinese customs and traditions; in doing so, Wang makes the reassuring discovery that his culture has provided almost most everything needed, technical expertise excepted, to provide good (read: Chinese) senior care.

While imaginary, this tale is drawn from my actual experiences; the characters are real and sourced from people I know and work with here in China. The story's various personalities are collected from a large circle of persons. They are at times merged to suit the narrative, my objectives and the less than perfect task of tale telling. The chronology is obviously compressed as well; the story begins at present day and extends about 7 years into an imaginary, but somewhat predictable, future.

My protagonist, Wang Xi, is a smart, practical man who can uncover the shortest route to a solution before most others understand the problem. He is a singular person who somehow escaped the die-cast, uniform molding that occurs in Chinese secondary education and developed a unique sense of individuality and self-determination. He is a Chinese capitalist with some heart and a good deal of soul. The story's antagonist is Huang Li; a self-important, petty, corrupt local municipal employee...enough said. The other characters are peripheral but supportive, lending color and tone to the sequence of events.

The politician

Wang grew frustrated with the local politician with whom he was speaking on his cell phone. The politician was a greedy weasel and Wang had already paid more than enough guanxi to obtain the reversal of land use rights so that he could sell apartments with title and not merely long term leases. Yet, the Weasel softly insisted that the approvals would be completed shortly if only Wang could provide additional financial assistance and show further appreciation for all the hard work on his behalf. Wang's cell phone was getting hot from use and his ear began to ache; he cursed the Weasel's mother under his breath. He paused to look out the tinted window of his new Bentley, and quickly crafted a solution to save both face, then proposed, "Huang Chu, I believe we each understand our respective challenges and should be able to help each other. I suggest we celebrate our mutual successes with a victory dinner next week. Do you think at this time we can enjoy ourselves and announce a final deal?" In an artfully simple yet firm statement, Wang conveyed his openness to Huang's suggestion but only for a final agreement. On the other end of the phone, the Weasel could barely contain his excitement; he complimented Wang on a thoughtful solution. When the Weasel got his way he usually gushed with delight and Wang had heard it all before. Chuckling, Wang smirked but thanked the Weasel. He turned his cell phone off and looked at Zhao Li, his long-time executive assistant and a trusted colleague, "It's done" he said quietly. "Take the necessary precautions, use a different transfer point…and Zhao Zong[44]…"

"Yes Sir?" Zhao responded attentively.

"Be careful, Huang is getting very greedy", Wang instructed.

"I will use an extra point of separation", Zhao faithfully reassured.

Of all the tasks Wang confronted in his business, payments such as these were distasteful to Wang. His style was more elementary; founded on substance. In somewhat of a very un-Han like characteristic, he was direct, yet, his frank manner had a beseeching grace. Nevertheless he participated in this warped system as this was the method and means.

Back at the City office, as Huang hung up he suggested to Wang they bring their close associates to an expensive new restaurant for the dinner. Huang was overjoyed with Wang's words and drew heavily on his cigarette; extracting yet more money from businessmen delighted him in a sensual way. As he exhaled broadly towards the ceiling, kicking his feet up onto his desk, he smiled with self-approbation and, speaking to an empty office, clapped his hands and sarcastically congratulated the rich developer on

---

44 Zong, Ju, Chu and Dong Ze Jiang are polite titles in Mandarin whose English equivalents are Director (business only), Bureau chief, Director and Chairman.

having secured his approvals. Huang shouted for his assistant to come into his office.

"Cheng Ju", Huang began to instruct. "Remember never let the developers dictate your responsibilities or pace of work....the approvals are ours to disperse and we deserve rich rewards for our hard work." Huang continued lecturing, "Now take these approval applications down to processing office and tell them the developer has met all the criteria for safety and employment conditions...get them signed this afternoon!"

Cheng Zhang was a dutiful assistant but a person with a bent toward reflection and one who found particular delight in sublime understatement; Huang's arrogance and corruption grated on him deeply. What's more Cheng found Huang an insufferable bore and disliked all the dinners he was required to attend at which he only listened to Huang boast of his power, accomplishments and the money he made vending his influence; not at all unlike the street hawkers peddling cheap fakes. Cheng saw these as ugly successes and hollow achievements. Cheng often reflected on the emptiness he felt working for Huang and the guilt that he felt processing the paid-for approvals. At heart, Cheng represented a new generation of Chinese bureaucrats. A more self-possessed and urbane class who sensed a responsibility to the municipality.

Cheng collected the Wang Xi documents and shuffled them neatly into a file. Before he left his 5th floor office for the processing department, Cheng paused and almost as an afterthought and possibly even as insurance, quietly made a 2nd copy of the Wang application and slipped it into his bottom desk drawer.

The hospital

Wang's driver aggressively pulled across traffic and into the driveway of People's Hospital #8 as oncoming traffic panicked and swerved to miss the expensive black car. The hospital was a hulking monstrous structure reminiscent of the architecture of Nuremburg; the building itself was also a reflection of the day which hung heavy in the grey smog of a late Beijing afternoon. Wang tossed his cell phone into his leather bag as his driver opened the door of the Bentley. He stepped out of the car and walked up the stairs, automatically without saying a word to his driver. The hospital lobby was a hive of activity; nurses running about with clipboards, patients' complaining about inattention, everyone seemed to present an obstacle to Wang's path and his destination of the 5th floor. Wang's stride was forced and grudging. As he pressed the elevator button, Zhao shuffled up to him and offered him a cell phone indicating it was an urgent call from Huang's office. Wang stepped into the elevator, turned and just shook his head as he pushed the 5th floor button; his mood for the Weasel had passed and could no longer tolerate small politicians. The elevator doors slid shut and for the first time that day Wang was alone; he breathed deep and mentally transported himself from work to his dying father.

The nurses on the 5th floor were dressed in dove-white uniforms. They expected Wang and as the elevator doors opened they flocked about him and dispensed words of consolation and hope. Half listening, Wang nodded in appreciation and asked for the doctor. He began the long walk down the hallway to the last room on the left which was always reserved for VIP's. It was a large room with a separate living room and bathroom, LED TV, stereo and exercise equipment. As Wang turned into his father's quarters from the corridor he paused and looked around, for the first time he wondered what all these useless extras had to do with his father's care.

As Wang approached his father he hardly recognized the man lying in the bed. In fact, Wang had never seen so many devices and thought it was hard to see him much less get close to him with all the machines surrounding the bed. It was like some tragic carnival, lights flashing, beeps and buzzing noises, tubes protruding painfully from his stomach. His father lay there unresponsive, resembling more a robot undergoing the replacement of some critical, mechanized component than the sweet old man Wang loved.

Wang stood there looking at his father confused and bewildered as the doctor hurried into the room. "Wang Dong Ze Jiang", the doctor said, "I am glad to see you. I regret to inform you that your father's condition is no better. My team and I are trying every possible modern treatment."

Wang turned and looked at the doctor, "Perhaps he is just an old, sick man, doctor...I am prepared to accept this and know that he will die."

"Never!" exclaimed the doctor. "We must always push our limits and try new ways" argued the doctor, in a vain attempt to both reassure Wang of his efforts and to justify the thick red envelope Wang had given him two weeks ago.

Wang surveyed the situation sensing its futility as well as the doctor's desperation. He responded calmly, "At what cost, Doctor? My father lies here dying like a machine....Where is the dignity in this? Why can't he die like a proud Han?"

The nurses stepped back feeling uncomfortable with the exchange between the doctor and Wang. The Doctor withdrew his opposition and became defensive, "I am a healer Chairman Wang. I am only trying to help your father."

Wang continued his advance, "It would appear that you are more mechanic…..Please leave me I want to be alone with my father."

"As you wish, Chairman", the Doctor bowed his head slightly and left the room with the nurses.

Wang's father had been unconscious for a week and was to die within a day. As Wang stood there he looked out the window and wondered how he….no…how they all…could have come to this point where parents are relegated to such care standards. Wang didn't so much question the overwhelming technical interventions of his father's treatment, as he did its lack of humanity. A cascade of memory flushed over Wang as he remembered his father caring for his grandmother 35 years ago. Wang recalled his grandmother, Wang Dai Yen, was nearly 100 years old when she passed. His father would spend hours away from work caring for his mother; washing her, feeding her, being a dutiful son. The memory caused a pang of guilt within Wang and brought a cleansing lucidity and he wondered for a moment about his path in life…he stood at one of life's chasm's…calculating the net value of his contribution to life and society as if the correct answer would brook safe passage over this frightening abyss. But he was not sure if all he had achieved to this point was equal to the challenge of this moment… he saw no clear bridge. But his native confidence supported him and he was certain that his Father's death would open up a new door and provide a crossing that would guide him to something much greater…and more important.

Wang stepped between one of the machines and the bed. He leaned over his father and stroked his head gently. As his fingers combed through his father's thick black hair, he whispered "Sleep well dear Baba, sleep now…"

In the weeks which followed, Wang seldom went to his office preferring instead his desk at home. He thought long and hard about his father's death, searching for some positive construct from the event. As he contemplated all his life's experiences, his instinct repeatedly brought him back to his duty to society. Wang remembered his father's admonition:

> *"In one's lifetime, one should fulfill one's responsibility in realizing the ideal of a harmonious society. Heaven relentlessly pursues its eternal movement, and a gentleman should make unremitting efforts to improve himself. If a man does what he can to fulfill his responsibility to life, at the moment of his death he will feel composed and have no qualms when he leaves this world."[45]*

Wang recognized these words as pure Confucian ideology and they were comforting. It gave him purpose in this life with death being no distraction. As he meditated, he considered his business and how he might further his own contribution to a harmonious society. Wang confronted himself: Have I set a fine example in virtue? Have I achieved a great career? And what have I to leave behind? His answers were incomplete and thus he knew he had a much longer road to travel and this future seemed inextricably linked to his father's death.

The dinner

Huang arrived at the restaurant early and eager to show off his new suit and shoes; he was ecstatic with himself...full of proportionless ego. Cheng reluctantly trudged along behind Huang and into the restaurant with a briefcase as Huang arrogantly ignored

---

45 This is something that Confucius said, I believe.

the Maître 'D and skipped straight to the VIP rooms. This was a singular night for Huang as he was able to triple his normal fee with the favors given to Wang, a very special evening indeed. He walked around the table deliberating the seating; he would place himself and Wang Xi directly next to one another; commensurate with each other's status, this would facilitate toasting each other and would allow Huang close conversation about other possible land parcels to which he had access. The rest of the dinner guests were superfluous.

Huang opened the private room's door and bellowed for a waitress. He wanted a menu. As he scanned through the listings of dishes, outside the restaurant Wang's car pulled up. Huang dictated the meal's dishes to the young woman and instructed her to ensure that the bottle

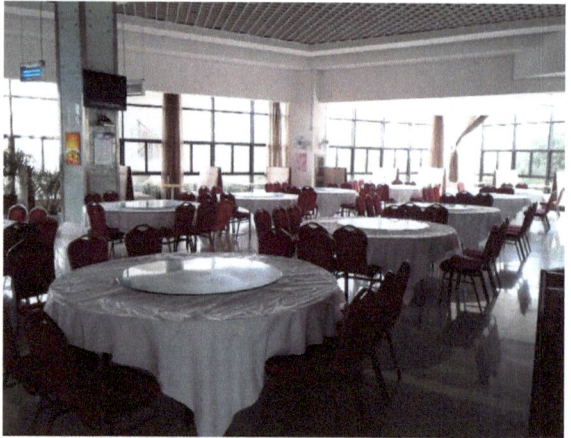

Figure 33 Dining room at Cherish Yearn, Pudong Shanghai

of Moutai was both genuine and fresh; tonight was much too important to brook a forgery.

In front of the restaurant, Wang's driver shifted the car into park and jumped from the driver's seat and rushed to open the far side passenger door. Wang was in a tight mood, stiff and focused; he was in no humor for delay or distraction. For Wang, tonight was a beginning; a place and time to end the dysfunctional relationship with Huang and begin a totally new episode in his construction business. With Zhao following close behind they marched into the restaurant. The Maitre 'D expected Wang and smiled as he entered. As Wang approached, the Maitre 'D leaned forward and whispered the room number where Huang was ensconced; it was one of the more expensive private rooms. Wang chuckled to himself and wondered if Huang would have such frequent luxury in the future.

Wang entered the dining room in full stride as Huang was speaking on his cell phone. Huang noticed Wang's stern demeanor as he hung up his phone but tried to ignore it. As he approached Wang he held out his arms expecting a ceremonial embrace.

"Wang Dong Ze Jiang", Huang announced. "Congratulations on your success!"

Wang coldly dismissed the attempt at polite embrace and held out his hand. "Huang Chu," Wang fired. "Thank you, but we haven't much time this evening....please sit".

At these words, Huang deflated. Wang's solemn mood cut deeply and severed Huang's elation. He knew something bad was about to happen. Cheng, frozen in the room's far corner, relished every moment of his boss's present demise, trying to calculate some play here for himself.

Sensing he had diminished Huang's ego to a proper size for a weasel, Wang moved to sit. Zhao brought Wang's briefcase and placed it alongside Wang on the table.

"Please, sit...Huang Chu. Let me tell you of the new plans." Wang said as he sat back in his chair he thought now was a good time to allow Huang a modicum of face. He opened the bottle of Moutai and poured Huang, and then himself, a drink.

Huang was perplexed and looked lost. He held out his hands in confusion as he sat. "Bu..but…," Huang stuttered.

"Huang Chu!" Wang barked then sipped his Moutai. "The market has changed…apartments are no longer easy money." I have made a decision to change the course and focus of my company."

Huang barely could absorb Wang words. He was still stuck on trying to understand how his dinner had gone from a triumph to catastrophe so fast? He looked at Wang bewildered; Huang was a shallow person and had no character on which to revert in moments such as these. Wang continued to command the situation and gave Huang a brief overview of his plans.

"Huang", Wang patronized, "You should be pleased as I am giving you the first news of this momentous decision. I am about to build a great company that will focus on care for our respected parents."

"Huh…excuse me?" Huang mumbled as he reached for the Moutai…another drink, he thought, would help him gather his mind.

"I am changing all operations from apartments to the building of senior living homes!" Wang declared with supreme confidence.

Huang swallowed a 3th jigger of fiery Moutai…Now looking at Wang with renewed confidence he inhaled deeply and responded, "But you know nothing of this business, Wang Dong Ze Jiang… why aren't you staying with what you do best…what about our partnership?"

Wang reached into his briefcase and pulled out some documents, instructing as he gave the papers to Huang, "Ah, Huang Chu, there is no need to discuss my motivations here…I doubt you would understand anyway. I trust that you will take these permits and renew them for my new elderly housing development."

With these words Wang was relieved that this was likely his last dealing with the Weasel. While his new venture would still require land and permits, the purpose for such would take him through different channels and higher venues who truly understood his altruistic endeavors. Huang poured himself another Moutai…the moment was completely lost on him.

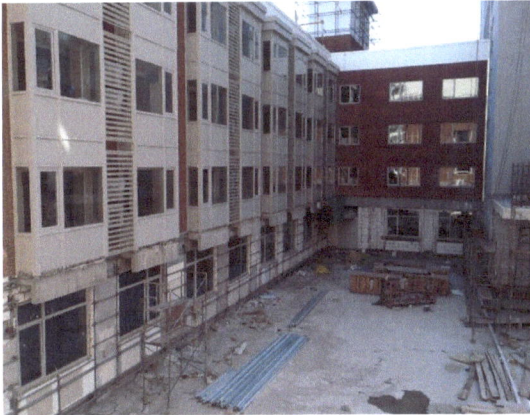

Figure 34 Yue Cheng (Landgent) facility in Beijing

Wang had neither the inclination nor the need to discuss with Huang his decision to turn his company into a senior living owner-operator. After all, it was more a personal decision than a business one anyway. Wang poured himself a sip of Moutai, raised it to Huang and drained it, showing his empty glass to Huang as he finished. Wang then stood up.

"Huang Chu….enjoy your dinner. Good night!

Wang turned and left with Zhao trailing silently behind him. Huang was left in the room alone but for a near empty bottle of Moutai and Cheng; Huang's good fortune had finally run dry.

Wang Xi's legacy

In the years after his father's death, Wang came to build no fewer than 35 facilities throughout China for seniors with a total of nearly 27,000 units. He built his new empire in a way that was not unlike the way he created his previous company, but it did differ in a few respects. First, Wang was smart enough to know he knew little of this new business. Sure, he was more than capable of erecting a building but he was equally smart enough to know what he didn't know. And in this case it was the day to day operations of a care facility. Second, he sensed that the opportunity in caring for this emerging demographic cohort wasn't confined to merely shelter and medical treatment but carried the promise of a much larger business which included selling the indirect necessities and support products for aging as well. Wang knew that the majority of older, wealthier Chinese were frugal and thrifty and they would eschew a costly new living environment preferring instead their own home. He surmised that the upper middle income cohort was the focus of a moderately priced senior living solution, not the mega rich. Besides, the mega-rich were relatively small in number and politically volatile.

Wang's innate sense of enterprise guided him well as did his exceptional resourcefulness. During the early years shortly after he had built his first two facilities, he was desperate for the knowledge and skills with which to operate the business. In this respect, he found nearly everything he needed through the attention of foreign companies eager to sell him long-dated management contracts. From these Lao Wai's[46], he asked and received many enthusiastic proposals of which he accepted none. These tenders contained great detail on what services needed to be performed and some information on how they should be performed. Of course Wang

---

46 Lao Wai is Mandarin for foreigner. Depending on context it can be mildly uncomplimentary to belittling.

knew that what he could learn from a proposal was not going to enable him operational proficiency, but it would provide him with a start and that's all he ever needed. From the proposals and the many attendant meetings, he and his newly hired staff listened attentively, gained a foothold and from there formulated a basic plan. As occupancy grew, they would then learn all that was needed. "Absorb all we can...learn as we go...teach ourselves...use our own Han instincts and our strong cultural teachings such as filial piety",...this was Wang's guiding mantra. And Wang was right for his purpose and his context, in fact, to foster continued family bonds between generations, Wang led the "inter-generational" housing style in China.

In all Wang had no interest in a Lao Wai running his facilities in a Western way and under a Western brand. Brands had limited appeal in this industry he reasoned...he could find no leading global senior living brand on which he could lever himself. Quite the contrary, he felt strongly...no, he *knew* that he could construct a Chinese brand on the back of Western technical knowhow. And that is what he did.

During his building of an operator, Wang naturally developed tangential businesses as well. In his efforts to build a modern medical staff, he also supported his client's occasional preference for Traditional Chinese Medicine treatments. This focus led Wang to create a whole line of traditional Chinese geriatric vitamins and health supplements. Likewise, he also appreciated certain Western geriatric products such as specialty beds, walkers and scooters so much he became an early distributor. But after time he grew disenchanted with the Lao Wai's profit split and manufactured the products himself using OEM specifications. In short, Wang became one of a few Kings of China Senior Living having used nothing more than his ingenuity, perseverance and a little borrowed expertise.

While in truth Wang's efforts to build an operator were indeed haphazard when compared to a present day Western approach, but in practicality this evaluation is unfair and almost irrelevant. What is important and pertinent is that his efforts were embraced and wholly accepted by those that mattered. It is true that some Western senior living businesses did flourish in China during these years but these successes were achieved over a very long period of time and at great cost. The more germane comparison here is the breadth of success Wang realized versus the achievements of Western companies during the same period of time.

Wang's accomplishments did not end there however. By 2025, China's global economic dominance gave Wang enormous confidence. And in a move of supreme irony and reversal of trends, he embarked on an enterprise to bring his traditional Chinese geriatric medicines, healing balms and care techniques to the West. He levered his brand off the mystique that surrounds Traditional Chinese Medicine and in time established a loyal and dedicated Western consumer following. After a few misfires, he even gained a surprising FDA approval for many of his treatments. His Western competitors were confounded by his abilities and despite their entreaties to discuss his methods, Wang never made business proposals; to do so would release his secrets. He preferred instead to be hired based on his record.

In the years following the apogee of Wang's business, he would often reflect on the three profound questions with which his father admonished him. It gave Wang great solace to finally see in quite a tangible way the virtue he had set, the success of his firm and the legacy would someday leave behind.

A final thought

For those of you who, like me, are constantly trying to understand the Chinese, I implore you to read as much Confucian philosophy as you can stand. It is a watershed of insight.

I leave you with this thought: Wen Tianxiang, a national hero in China's history, wrote the following on his belt just prior to his execution:

> *"Confucius teaches benevolence and Mencius teaches righteousness. For the sake of righteousness, perfect benevolence could be attained. What else can a man learn from the sages? After my death, I will feel no qualms at all."*

In the final analysis, much of Chinese thought on life and death (although Confucius does not discuss death much preferring instead to concentrate on life) can be distilled within the Confucian ideal that, should a person fulfill his social responsibility before death, he will die "immortal." In his venture into senior living, Wang inhabited this ideal creating a Chinese solution for a Chinese challenge.

Intermission: Oh, Shandong...I Long To See You...
中场片段: 啊山东...期待相遇

The history of Shandong province is, in more ways than one, a recapitulation of China's history which, at least for the last 200 years, is a story predominately about its relationship with the West. Quite a lot of what happened in China either began here or involved Shandong in some way or another. And while Shandong has played

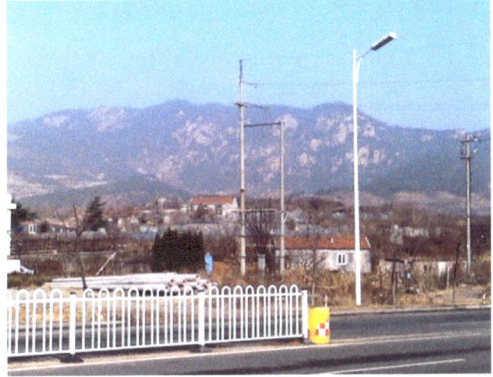

Figure 35 Future location in Qingdao for 25,000 senior apartments set on 10,000 acres

an important part of the cultural development of China since antiquity (from Qi State to Qin Period and through the Han, Jin, Sui, Tang and Song Dynasties) the area was not formalized as a province until the Ming Dynasty. It wasn't until the Qing and rule under the Manchus in 1644 that it assumed its current boundaries as occupying all of the Shandong Peninsula (and part of East-Central China) separating the Bohai Bay from the Yellow Sea. Another interesting fact of Shandong is that it can claim, among the more important persons who were born and lived in the province, Confucius. No one has, arguably, impacted Chinese culture and thought more than he. Today, Shandong and its principal commercial city, Qingdao (although Jinan is the provincial capital) are fully modernized urban centers and have populations of 9.5 million and nearly 9 million[47], respectively.

---

47 Qingdao is the second most populous city in Shandong after Linyi whose population is over 10 million.

Shandong has a long and hard relationship with foreign influence. Following a suite of concessions to foreign governments elsewhere in China, in 1896 the unraveling Qing Dynasty leased much of Shandong (except Weihai which was leased to the British) to the Germans who established their headquarters in Qingdao. Shortly afterwards, the Boxer Rebellion, born in Shandong, launched a bloody assault on foreigners in China. The Boxers, or more formally the Society of Righteous and Harmonious Fists, was a secret society consisting largely of local farmers/peasants and other workers made desperate by disastrous floods, famines and widespread opium addiction. Rightly or wrongly, they laid the blame on Christian missionaries (protected from local law under extraterritoriality), Chinese Christians, and the Europeans colonizing their country.

The Boxers originated from the Lí sect of the Ba Gua religion group. Foreigners came to call the well-trained, athletic young men "Boxers" due to the martial arts and calisthenics they practiced. The Boxers' other notable trait was spirit possession, which involved "the whirling of swords, violent prostrations, and chanting incantations to Taoist and Buddhist spirits."[48] The Boxers believed that through training, diet, martial arts, and prayer they could perform super human feats, such as flight. Further, they popularly claimed that millions of spirit soldiers would descend from the heavens and assist them in purifying China of foreign influences. The legacy of the Boxers has no doubt contributed greatly, if not in whole, to the fantastic Wuxia martial arts movie genre; a staple of the Chinese cinematic experience. Eventually the Rebellion was put down and many of the Boxers and their government counterparts were executed.

---

48 This information on the Boxers was sourced from Wikipedia.

And if the German occupation[49] and the Boxer Rebellion weren't enough turmoil, as a consequence of the German loss in World War 1, the Treaty of Versailles extinguished the German Shandong concession and granted occupation to Japan providing them an excellent logistics headquarters for their future aggression in China.

In all, Qingdao has a bit of a sad history but while its past has been quite tumultuous, today, Qingdao is experiencing a rebirth as if it is receiving a bountiful payback for all its past suffering under both foreign as well as cruel, internal dynastic rule. Recently, it played a smart role in China's

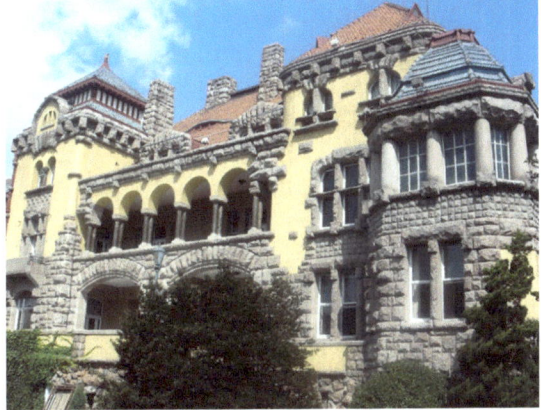

Figure 36 German Governor's mansion, Qingdao (Wkpd)

2008 Olympic debut hosting the sailing competitions and displaying many of the city's world class, highly westernized attributes. The province is indeed among the most productive and richest in China.

Yet, this renaissance may not be entirely in Qingdao's best interest. In much of Shandong, not just Qingdao, unrestrained industrialization has spoiled much of the natural rocky-hills beauty that was once the inspiring backdrop of many its local cities. Intense real estate development has raked the landscape so thoroughly as to denude it of any soul; it's beautiful hills blown

---

49 In comparison with the Japanese occupation, one can convincingly argue that the Germans provided the province of Shandong and their headquarters in Qingdao with quite a bit more civic benefits, including a sanitary supply of drinking water, a rarity for Asia in the early 1900's. Nearly as notable, they also built the Germania Brewery which after expropriation by the Communists became the Tsingtao Brewery.

apart with dynamite then plowed flat to create additional land for office buildings, commercial centers and towering apartment buildings. The foreign influences the Shandongese fought against so fervently for so long are today fully ingrained in their daily lives; on some level they have become what they hated. There are 4 super high end car dealerships in Qingdao, among them Bentley and Lamborghini…KFC's are more available than noodle shops… and everyone wears Armani.

Song of Shandong

Every morning around 10am in the old city of Qingdao, on the corner of Xinhu Lu and Dongtinghu Lu an elderly man, lonely and forlorn, appears from a side alley on his way to sit in the shade of the intersection's only Willow tree; he

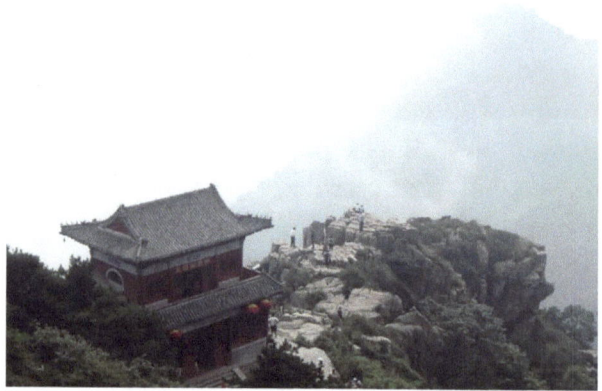

Figure 37 Mount Tai, Shandong (Wkpd)

looks 100 years old. He walks up to the corner, ducks under the tree's branches and slowly unfolds a stool. Once seated, he peers up and down the street as if looking for someone; takes a breath and settles himself. Gazing up into the tree and marveling at its beautiful green canopy, he pauses and begins a mournful chant; his eyes are shut. When I first heard it, I was reminded of the old American folk song Oh Shenandoah! whose melancholy words and pensive music make one yearn for home and a time that once was.Though the old man's voice is deep and low, every word seems to rise effortlessly from his lips up into the Willow's branches, drifting towards heaven. It is an epic, remorseful song of how things once were in Shandong; a narrative his grandfather taught him a time long ago. His grandfather, in turn, was taught the melody by his grandfather and it tells a tale of a time before the rush by greedy Europeans and impetuous Japanese to snatch up imperial possessions…when Qingdao was a quiet fishing village populated by extended families. It is a soulful, nostalgic tune full of paradise lost. A song of homesick fishermen eager to return from sea with their catch to wives and children back in beautiful Shandong, of strict monastic dedication to the tenets of Buddhism and righteous espousal of Taoism and of now, saddest of all…that none of this world exists any longer and is replaced with something that only superficially resembles what Shandong used to be. When listening to him one understands how unmoored his generation feels in today's Shandong; adrift in a tempest of modernity,

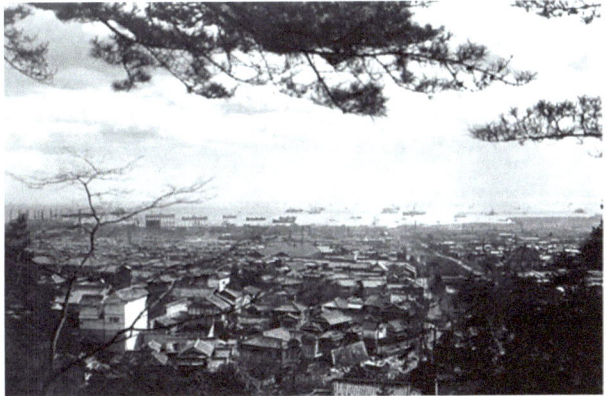

Figure 38 German occupied Qingdao circa 1912 (www.cityofart.net)

submerged below the surface of society and now lost beyond the horizon of Qingdao's consciousness. When the old man finishes his song, he just sits there quietly for a while gathering himself. The late Qingdao morning traffic screams through the intersection, its unbearable cacophony almost shouting him out of existence. Soon he picks himself up, folds his stool, steps out from under the Willow and heads back down the alley. After a minute he is gone and, like the times of which he sings, nearly forgotten. When he finally passes on, these memories will likely disappear permanently and Qingdao becomes the lesser for it.

Before I left the intersection where he sang, I asked a young lady dressed in smart designer outfit hurrying past me on her way to work who the old man was. She chuckled cynically and with a brush of her hand dismissed my inquiry as a waste of her time. "Just some crazy old man", she said. For the word "crazy" she uses a derisive Mandarin term for dementia. As she turned away, a zhong from a nearby Buddhist temple reverberated with a low, thunderous timbre. At that precise moment, watching as the young woman fought her way back into the crowd, I thought to myself, "Ask not for whom the bell tolls, it tolls for you." I later learned that the old man has no more family so he sings to anyone who will listen; of course few do.

It is clear the Shandongese have little time to waste on silly old tales; though knowing where things have been might help them understand where things are going. As one might expect, old German occupation-era pictures of Qingdao show quite a different scene than what one experiences today; 100 years ago it was a pretty city by the sea with a bustling port, getting busier by the day. Few of the buildings constructed then still exist and sadly, even less of the traditional lifestyle survives. What was once the serene province of Confucius and no doubt a hub of quiet, contemplative daily life is a distant memory remembered only in faded old photographs and in the songs of crazy old men.

DementiaTown
觉 醒 痴 眠 城

"You may think you know what you're dealing with,
but believe me, you don't."
Water baron Noah Cross in **_Chinatown_**

Dementia is the tragedy that keeps on giving; like an irreversible decree of solitary confinement for an innocent man, growing increasingly confused and distraught by the day, he slowly goes mad while his family, helpless and heartbroken, stands by and watches his decline. Sure, some medications can alleviate, alternative therapies can relieve, but the painful truth is that these are temporary and superficial; in the long run those so diagnosed are simply doomed to a long, slow, costly cognitive degeneration unwinding into an inevitable, undignified death. That's dementia.

The confusing thing about dementia is that there are many different types: Alzheimer's, Vascular Dementia, Fronto-temporal Dementia, Parkinson's, Huntington's, Creutzfeldt-Jakob, Wernicke-Korsakoff and others. What's more unsettling is that each variation of the disease offers its victim a special hell: extreme paranoia, hyper anxiety, hallucinations, depression, hostility, inability to reason. In my opinion, the disease ranks high among the worst plagues - smallpox, typhus, Ebola and cholera; it is indiscriminate and unmerciful. Professionally, I have been around dementia patients to some extent and I still need to steel myself when touring a facility. Dementia care professionals must be among the toughest, most heroic people (along with NICU nurses) on earth.

Dementia has been around forever but it wasn't identified (in the particular case of Alzheimer's) until 1906 when a German physician named Dr. Alois Alzheimer, specifically identified a collection of brain cell abnormalities as a disease. One of Dr. Alzheimer's patients died after years of severe memory problems, confusion and difficulty understanding questions. Upon her death, Dr. Alzheimer performed a brain autopsy, and noticed dense deposits surrounding the nerve cells. Inside the nerve cells he observed unusual, twisted bands of fibers. Today, this degenerative brain disorder bears his name, and when found during an autopsy, these plaques and tangles mean a definite diagnosis of Alzheimer's disease. Today, we know enough about dementia so we don't really need to wait until after death to confirm a diagnosis, but autopsies are invaluable from a scientific/research point of view.

Chongqing People's Hospital #45

In downtown Chongqing there sits on a crowded street a large grey concrete hospital generically called People's Hospital #45. PH45, as I will refer to it, is not a large hospital but it is clean and enjoys a good reputation among its patrons. Its patrons, curiously, are relatively well off financially as they are high ranking members of the local government or military personnel. PH45 is a privileged-patient hospital, the poor or middle class Chinese are not served. Why is this?... one asks the natural question while in the largest communist country in the world? Why would the harmonious society ideal impose such inequality, not to mention hypocrisy, on its dutiful citizens especially when it comes to such a basic human need such as health care? Ah, this is China and contradictions are a way of life. One quickly learns after spending some time here that China is one of the most class segmented societies on earth...another blatant "contradiction-as-way-of-life" aspect to this fascinating country. Let's move on.

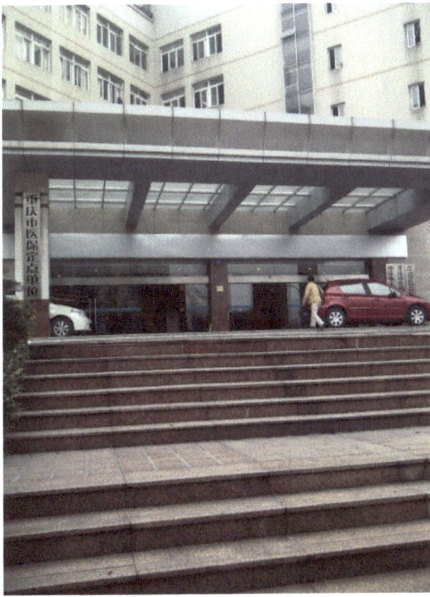

Figure 39 Long Hu Hospital, Chongqing

PH45 is a hospital that, to my somewhat informed eye, is a good facility; fairly clean, busy and like I mentioned earlier, it seems to have good status. There are about 600 total beds dispersed over 9 floors; the hospital claims "heart treatments" as its specialty. But during our visit, my destination was the 7th floor which I understood was entirely devoted to geriatric care and indeed it is. My staff arranged for a Tour guide in advance and when we arrived at PH45, a non-descript young lady of about 30 years old was waiting for us. Li Xi was her name.

The 7th floor

One exits the elevators into a very crowded lobby consisting of about 25 square meters. There is a reception counter, two cheap white plastic chairs (poolside variety), and a lonely, fake house plant sitting on top of a white plastic table (also poolside) and numerous brown cartons of some consumer product stacked up against the walls. The overall impression is of sterile, cold utilitarianism.

Our tour guide introduces us briefly to a giggling receptionist...she is a young woman who is wearing a pink tee-shirt with the image of a playboy bunny on the front imprinted with silver sequins; the image bears the caption "I'm a fun bunny!" We all smile and nod.

Just as we complete this routine, the Chief Nurse arrives on scene to meet us. Nurse Rang Chek greets us solemnly (my over-active imagination kicks in immediately indexing her from the sound of the name…Ah! She's Nurse Ratched from *One Flew Over The Cuckoo's Nest*…the coincidence is both amusing and creepy at the same time). She is a short but a powerfully stout woman, unyielding, methodical; a battlefield nurse well-versed in medical triage, I imagine to myself. We exchange pleasantries but I can tell Nurse Ratch…I mean Rang Chek, is suspicious; wondering what these Lao Wai's are doing in her hospital. Just in case, Nurse Rang Chek beckons for two assistants to escort us on the tour; the message: there will be *no* Randle McMurphy style insurrection here.

The main corridor for the 7th floor runs perpendicular to the lobby and elevator doors. There are 12 patient rooms and a shocking 66 occupied beds, half of which are littered about the hallway, a few in the reception and 2 in what used to be the nurse's restroom. It was seized from nursing use when overcrowding reached its present state. We began our tour by turning left out of the lobby down one half of the hallway.

The first 10 beds which we pass in the corridor are occupied by sleeping patients whose average age, I guess, is around 85. They are wizened old men and women with sunken cheeks and large blue veins scoring their pale arms. Each of them has multiple iv's stuck into the back of their wrists.

"Can you tell me the primary diagnosis of the patients here is?", I inquire of Li Xi.

Li Xi responds in a Mandarin phrase I am not familiar with and I ask my staff what she said.

"Old age sickness", my staff responds.

"Old age sickness?" I ask quizzically, "What is that?"

There is a dialogue between my staff, Li Xi and me that seems to be half negotiation and half interpretation. In the end it is agreed by all that most of the patients have some sort of cancer, recent major surgery or have 痴呆 or its English equivalent, dementia. Through a little deduction and further persistent inquiry, I surmise that there must be at least 20 patients at PH45 with dementia.

We pass by an elderly woman, a dementia patient, fast asleep on her bed in the hallway. She has a sweet face and beautiful fiery white, wild hair. I look at Li Xi and ask her why nearly every patient we have seen is sleeping. She responds quickly with absolute confidence in her answer, "Their sickness makes them very sleepy, so they sleep most of the time." Li Xi smiles at me, beaming broadly at having known the answer so well and quickly.

I pause for a moment at the bed of the sweet old woman. I look at her and wonder. Just as I begin to contemplate her fate, she suddenly opens her eyes and glares directly at me. Startled, I leap back. She raises her hand and points an angry, accusing finger at me...I glance away and notice my staff has moved on ahead of me. Somewhat embarrassed at having the old woman catch me staring at her, I smile at her and quickly move on. But before I completely leave her side, I glance at her chart. Among others, her medications include large doses of Risperdal and Xanax.

My eyes widen in horror as I step back from the bed, I turn walk away from her and rejoin my staff. The rest of the tour is perfunctory and just more and more of the same: sedated patients, doing time, wasting away. And after an hour, my team and I graciously thank our proud Tour guide, compliment her on an excellent facility and escape to a bar down the street.

I take a long gulp from my glass of red wine. "So, comrades", I begin with some levity to chat with my staff. "What do we make of this place?"

I get blank stares.

"Ok, I will go first", I quip. I'm not sure if they are tired or shell-shocked like me.

I begin again, "Tell me guys, are the patients on the 7th floor being overly sedated because 1) the way Chinese hospitals make money is to prescribe drugs or 2) they don't know how to handle a demented, hostile old woman so they sedate her 24/7?".

"Both" my staff responds in unison as they now take a drink from their glasses.

I look at them in disbelief and confess, "I was afraid you would say that."

Dementia in China

There are no official numbers for the prevalence of dementia or any of its multiple forms in China which reflects both the lack of research as well as cultural stereotypes about the disease. But some time ago, Alzheimer's Disease International (ADI) published a report titled _The prevalence of dementia worldwide[50]_ in which it is estimated that 1.7% of the population of China (and its immediate

---

50 "The prevalence of dementia worldwide", ADI, December 2008, London UK. See www.alz.co.uk

neighbors) aged 65-69 have some sort of dementia rising to 3.7% for those aged 70-74. These figures grow dramatically to 7% for those in the 75-79 age cohort and double to 14.4% for those aged 80-84. ADI further estimated that for those aged 85 and older, 26.2% of the population has some incidence of dementia. Applying these percentages to 2008 population data indicates a (2008) total potential population with some level/form of dementia of **12.9 million** persons. Of course this figure is, in all likelihood, larger today by about 6% (the growth of China population since 2008). Another reputable source, WHO, pegs the total number of Chinese with dementia between **15 million** and **17 million**. This count seems somewhat within reason from a proportions point of view between the US[51] and China; but only if one believes dementia's prevalence is without regard to race or geography. Still another source of information, the China Alzheimer's Project[52] based in Beijing, estimates over **10 million** Chinese are afflicted with some form of Dementia. I have never attempted estimates for the total number of dementia afflicted persons in China and therefore can offer no other authority to substantiate these estimates. So, reader, take these on faith until I can support or establish otherwise.

For a country with not much in the way of advanced dementia treatment, these is are alarming figures to say the least especially when in many parts of China, mental illness is still viewed as a contagion. It is tantamount to a family embarrassment and those afflicted are shunned. Reports from caregivers and nursing homes in Beijing, Shanghai, Xi'an and elsewhere are rife with stories of newly admitted patients having been subjected to inhumane treatment, frequent abuse, incarceration or other sadistic behavior in their past. All is not lost, though...in fact the future is bright.

---

51 Estimates on the number of persons afflicted with dementia in the US approach 5 million.

52 See http://www.memory360.org/en/

From my experience and the experiences of a few Japanese and Western dementia professionals who have traveled to China and with whom I have spoken, we can collectively report an insatiable craving on the part of Chinese "mental health" professionals to learn more about the disease and how to effectively treat it without excessive reliance on anti-psychotic drugs to sedate. There is an overt eagerness to understand, learn and treat; an encouraging and hopeful start. In sum, within the context of China's greater senior living/geriatric consumables opportunity, I firmly believe dementia treatments, represent yet another great opportunity for knowledgeable technicians from both charitable (IP imparting) as well as a business, profit driven imperative points of view. Nevertheless, Noah Cross's fateful rebuke to JJ Gittes in *Chinatown* regarding his lack of knowledge about the investigation[53] is as true for the Chinese as it is for their Western peers when it comes to dementia; the disease is a stubborn mystery.

As a final note, many in the West refer to dementia treatment as "memory care" or another soft adjective which is supposed to make this whole subject less threatening, especially to the families of patients; and it may indeed. I didn't do that here as I think my audience is a more clinical readership who doesn't require such silk-tongued language when discussing the subject among professional counterparts.

Chinatown

Roman Polanski's last film in the US before becoming a fugitive from justice and fleeing to Europe was *Chinatown*[54]. The film, sort of a neo film-noir classic, is set in Los Angeles in 1937 and tells

---

53 Reference to initial quote in this essay "You may think you know what you are dealing with..."

54 Screenplay by Robert Towne

the tale of the bitter California water wars. The film was released in 1974 and ranks among the best movies ever made; it contains a little of everything: romance, tragedy, conspiracy, murder, mystery and street justice or injustice depending on your taste. The film stars an attractive cast: a very young and sly Jack Nicholson, splendid silver screen beauty Faye Dunaway and one of the greatest actors of all time, John Huston, whose portrayal of water baron Noah Cross (Noah...great name for a man in the business of water)...as a sociopathic, ruthless businessman is nothing short of brilliant. I love this film.

So what does Polanski's film *Chinatown* have to do with dementia in China? Nothing really...which is all well and good as I don't want to attempt making a larger point here than the story should carry. What's more, having seen the film a number of times I would really have to stretch metaphors to even come close to some meaningful allegory (although there is an assisted living home scene which gives an insight into early "Rest homes" in the US as well as a bit of religious bigotry). I just liked the way the movie's name "Chinatown" gave a way to link my experience on the Mainland with our visit to the 7th floor at PH45. Pouring it all into a story on www.ChinaSeniorLiving.com *and* staying consistent with artfully re-arranging Chinese-themed film titles really made it work for me. I would, however, like to point out that Polanski made a movie who's title *Chinatown* neither illuminates nor informs on the plot or the underlying whirlpool of California's water wars, so in turn, I feel somewhat licensed to use *DementiaTown;* after all what's in a title except for a little madness?

Vintery, mintery, cutery, corn,
Apple seed and apple thorn,
Wire, briar, limber lock
Three geese in a flock

**One flew East
One flew West
And one flew over the cuckoo's nest.**

-Early American children's nursery rhyme (anonymous)

Intermission: *NEWSFLASH* Fujian Elderly Jump Over The Tu Lou!
中场片段: 福建佛跳土楼

Geographically, Fujian Province is the navel in China's round belly. Located on the southeastern seaboard directly opposite Taiwan, it is about the same size as New York but it has a population of 39 million, twice that of the Empire state. Fujian is one of the most culturally and linguistically diverse provinces in China, due entirely to migration over the centuries. Ethnic peoples from all over the mainland flocked to the province not just to escape wars, but for the simple fact that it is a beautiful country with a very agreeable climate not unlike South Carolina. There is also abundance of China's special level 3 hospitals and for these reasons and more, it is perfect for retirees.

Among the Fujian immigrants were the Hakka, an ethnicity that originated in northern China and who settled in the southern provinces. From the 17th century onwards, population pressures drove them more and more into conflict with their neighbors. As this rivalry for resources turned

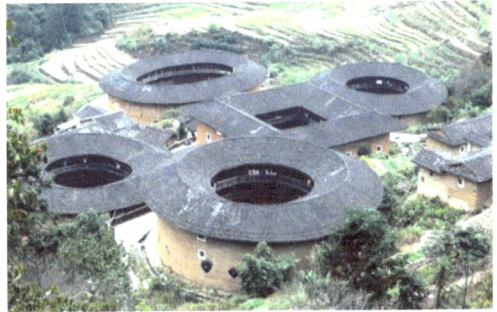

Figure 40 Tu Lou for Hakka people in Fujian (Martin Tai)

to armed warfare, the smart Hakka began designing their homes as easily defended forts (high walls and a single entrance) not to mention self-sufficient with independent water sources. These house-forts, called Tu Lou 土楼, were often round in shape and internally divided into many compartments for food storage, living quarters, ancestral temple, armory etc. Most importantly however, when one walks around inside a Tu Lou the communal feeling one gets is remarkable. In fact, with some modern improvements, the design looks like a great concept for assisted living or even dementia care.

Certainly the Province's beautiful weather, dramatic vistas and interesting local architecture are alluring but there is yet another reason to go to Fujian; namely their food. I highly recommend Fujian cuisine, and specifically, one dish in particular known as *Buddha-jumps-over-the-wall*. However odd the

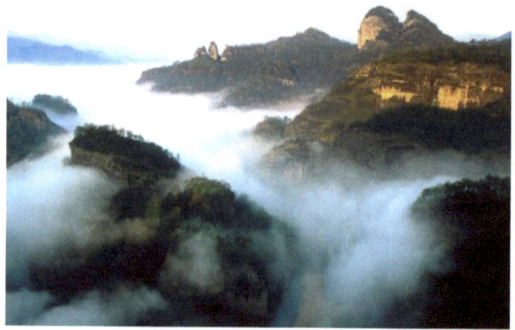

Figure 41 Vista in Fujian Province (China Travel)

name, it is delicious stew with an equally interesting history. As the story goes, during the Qing Dynasty a wise scholar was traveling by foot with his friends. As he trekked he preserved all his food for the journey, mixing it together indiscriminately, in a clay jar previously for holding wine. Whenever he was hungry, he heated the jar containing all the ingredients over an open fire. After one particularly long day's sojourn, the group arrived in Fuzhou, Fujian's capital. As the fire under the clay jar began to boil his food, the scent caught a gentle breeze and wafted over to a nearby Buddhist monastery where solemn monks were dutifully meditating. But while monks are not allowed to eat meat, the delectable fragrance was so irresistible that one of the monks couldn't resist the temptation. In a full frenzy, the monk leaped over the monastery's walls and zealously sought out the source of the aroma. Astonished at what he had just witnessed, one of the scholar's companions, a poet, immediately wrote down the recipe and claimed that it was so enjoyable that even a Buddha would scale a monastery's walls to eat the delicious dish.

Buddha-jumps-over-the-wall is a soup or kind of Chinese stew which contains many ingredients including quail eggs, bamboo shoots, scallops, abalone, shark fin, chicken, ham, pork tendon, ginseng, mushrooms, and taro. Cooking *Buddha-jumps-over-the-wall* takes a while...a few days of simmering at least. Certain of the ingredients, including the Shark's fin must be cooked on the first day and allowed to boil for some time with most of the other ingredients including the vegetables being added in just before serving. The final product is very tasty not unlike a western style gumbo, just not as thick. And eating *Buddha-jumps-over-the-wall* is an experience, because there are so many different items in the soup, each spoonful offers a delicious surprise.

The odd thing about Fujian, given all their positive and accommodating attributes for retirement living, to wit: healthy food, pleasant environment, intriguing architecture, etc., is that they don't have many senior living residences other than the government sponsored variety. One would think that someone would have figured this out by now, but they haven't.

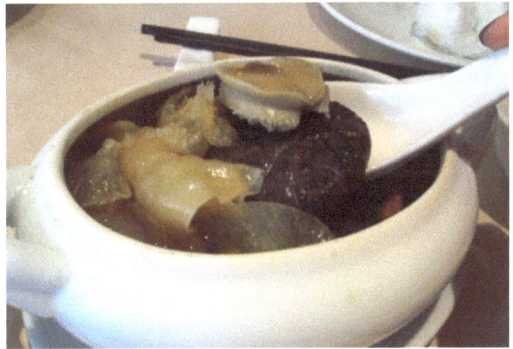

Figure 42 My Buddha-jumps-over-the-wall

Then again maybe there is a reason. What would they do with all these geriatric patients climbing the walls of the Tu Lou senior living facilities for a taste of mouthwatering Fujian stew being slow cooked just outside the gates…?

Eat, Drink (or absorb)…Geriatric Nutrition!
饮食滋人 关怀润心

"…my food is only as good as the expression on your face."
Master Chef Chu speaking to his best friend Old Wen in
Eat, Drink, Man, Woman

In this essay, I am less concerned with China than with another thing, namely the nexus of food, ageing and what the future may bring with respect to both. At the intersection of these three parallel themes there is a point of union which reveals just how far we are capable of transcending our humanity, if at all. And on the lighter side…could there be a better time of year to be talking about food than the week prior to Thanksgiving[55]?

This is the second time in the short history of this blog that I have channeled the work of Director Ang Lee. It turns out that he has an exceptional talent for harvesting raw human feeling, extracting sensitive experience…purifying it further with the essence of sympathetic understanding and then serving it to us revealing our own deeply held insecurities; his works are a hearty meals of therapy for the emotionally famished.

Lee's film *Eat, Drink, Man, Woman* (1994) is a full course meal full of spicy conflicts within a Chinese family, using food as a delicious metaphor for caring and a conduit to overcome familial relationship inadequacies. Master Chef Chu is a long-time widower who spends hours cooking large Sunday dinners for his three daughters Jia-Chien, Jia-Jen and Jia-Ning; all of whom have difficulty communicating their love for one another. For Chu, food is a means of expression, not only of his creativity but also of the

---

55 Obviously, this was written shortly before Thanksgiving 2012.

feelings of love and affection that he can't otherwise articulate. Food is his way of reaching out, of connecting; and in his constantly changing world, Chu nourishes in the only way he can, feeding the heart, soul as well as body of those he loves. As Chu feeds, he rises above his mortality; and in a sweet twist of fate that closes the movie in a beautifully heartfelt way, Chu regains his sense of taste while sharing a meal his daughter compassionately cooked only for him. He is in a word, inspirational.

While, regrettably, to live is to age; the regenerative and nourishing power of caring through measured sustenance cannot be underestimated. When prepared not just as a science experiment or by a contracted, indifferent caterer but as a calling and with the devotion an artist has for his canvass, I believe food can suspend, however temporary,

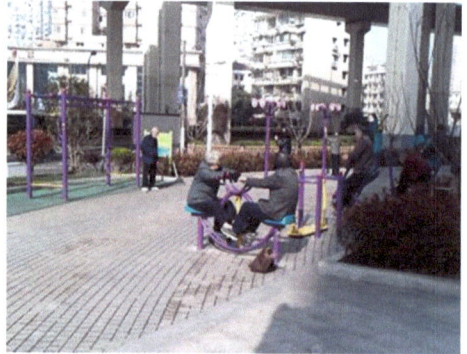

Figure 43 Shanghai elderly limber up at community exercise equipment

the less desirable aspects of ageing thus improving life. Yet for all the enhanced diets, all the attempts to enrich taste and arouse appetites, it seems to me that (cost aside) motivation is the single most critical issue frustrating geriatric nutritionists. And by motivation I mean encouraging the infirm to eat; inspiring a despondent elderly man who has long suppressed his hunger, to take a bite of his vegetables; stimulating an old woman with Alzheimer's who has lost her sense of taste to sit and have a meal; calmly, confidently and compassionately reassuring the aged who no longer recognize food as nourishing, that eating is indeed necessary. Ageing is complicated, and therefore the issues surrounding the sustenance of the elderly are naturally complex. I live and work in the senior care industry and presently live in China where geriatrics and gerontology has just been born... consequently the field of geriatric nutrition is really only an informal conversation among a handful of practitioners today. With its imminent demographic calamity, China lacks a defined geriatric nutrition which underscores not just the urgent need to develop a Chinese geriatric diet but to further understand all things geriatric in Chinese context.

Hors d'oeurves

It is universal that geriatric nutrition is or should be concerned primarily with two questions: First, what diet, begun in earlier years under frequent supervision and modification as the body changes, is conducive to a long and healthier life? And, second, what should be the diet of those already elderly?

Conventional wisdom dictates that the elderly must consume foods that are nutrient dense. It seems to me that identifying those food stuffs is only half the challenge; maintaining a nutritional balance (and further defining that balance) is the other, especially with an institutionalized elderly person. Further complicating are issues such as immobility, either in bed or in a chair, which contributes to a whole host of negative side effects including low nitrogen and pressure ulcers. So in order to offset such adverse conditions, one must provide enough dietary protein to maintain tissue integrity, muscle mass and immune function. There is, however, an erroneous assumption by many health care practitioners that elderly people cannot tolerate large amounts of dietary protein because of their renal function. But in the absence of extensive renal disease, I understand most elderly people can tolerate high levels of dietary protein if they are adequately hydrated.

The above is all good and well, sounds practical and well informed. And I am sure that, after some long and focused study, some meaningful Chinese dietetic counterpart would and will still emerge. After all, so much of traditional Chinese food is healthy not to mention delicious; the recent spike in diabetes and obesity being entirely attributable to the loss of customary foodstuffs, an increase in fast food, sugary carbonated drinks and other western, highly sought after snacks.

But the more I think about the whole concept of geriatric nutrition, I wonder if it isn't a fleeting construct that could and may very well be replaced in due time with another more modern, more technologically enhanced diet; a designer-diet that has been purposefully engineered to stave off disease and reduce cellular degeneration. Perhaps in the near future, the diet of not just older persons but people of all ages becomes, just as an osteopathic surgeon replaces an old man's knees with a mechanical joint

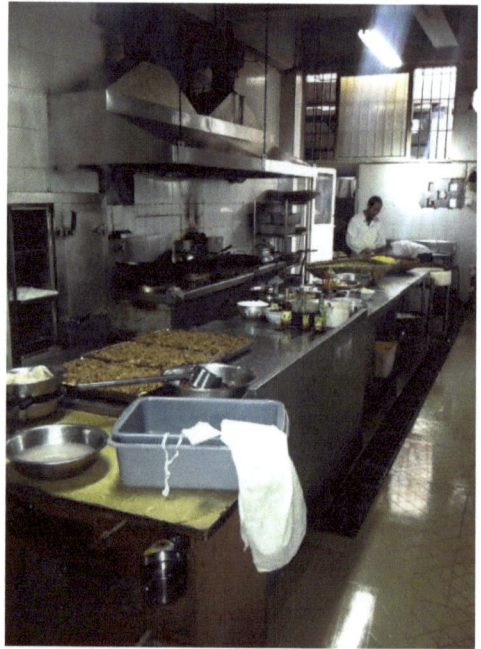

Figure 44 Kitchen facility at Guihou Senior Living, Chongqing

made of space age Teflon (which is in many ways an improvement over his original), simulated nourishment; micro-meals delivered in pill form or skin patches and absorbed into the epidermis. Their molecular constituencies would be programed to seek out metabolic deficiencies and deliver measured doses of certain foodstuffs, drugs or vitamins. In some ways this concept is already with us (to wit: nicotine patches). Maybe there is a "nutritional singularity" in the sense that Ray Kurzweil used the word in his 2005 novel *"The Singularity Is Near"*.

I would like to, for the duration of this essay, suspend a typical dialogue about food, diet and what may or may not be acceptably nutrient dense and explore a competing vision of what the future may bring with respect to nourishment. Where are we headed and what will food look like in 50 years? I wonder if geriatric nutrition will even be a concern…

A lazy-susan daydream

A group of friends and I exited the movie theatre located off Fuxing Lu in downtown Shanghai and carefully made our way across the busy intersection to a senior living facility whose name I have changed to Wing-on. The movie, *Eat, Drink, Man, Woman* had left us all, quite understandably, very hungry, and we were eager to take advantage of an invitation to dine with the elderly residents of Wing-on.

The dining hall at Wing-on is not optimally situated within the Wing-on campus but hidden on the far side of the property forcing elderly residents into a long, hungry march. All 6 of us trekked across the sinuous walkways as a cold mid-November wind blew across the campus. We reached the cafeteria chilled and even more famished than before. We all sat down at a large round table on heavy, bulky wooden chairs which require a fair amount of strength and agility to maneuver. We did not order any food but instead, simply received the prescribed meal for that day prepared by a cadre of workers: landing on the table were bowls of white rice, a sweet/sour spare rib dish, steamed bok-choy in an oily, garlic sauce, whole broiled fish (yes: head, bone and fin intact) a non-descript broth in which random pieces of meat (chicken?) were floating, a sesame-seed cake/pastry with a sweet red bean filling for dessert and of course, rivers of tea (Longjing) to wash it all down. Most of this food I have had before here in China, it is good and tasty. But I have not the slightest idea whether or not it is "nutrient dense" or that it contains any of the important things the elderly really need; I strongly suspect no one does. But it is what is served at Wing-on and what the residents have eaten for their entire lives…it seems to make them happy.

As our group began to dig in to the meal, residents of Wing-on began to enter the cafeteria, happily chatting about all sorts of things from their Mahjong game earlier to a highly anticipated marriage of a grandson. They all seemed a content crowd as they lined up, buffet style to collect trays and receive helpings of that day's meal…

Bromme 柯博明: I am glad we all could make this meal. I have been thinking a great deal lately about what is happening not just in China today but the plight of the ageing globally. In the context of the movie we just had and now eating where we are, I thought each one of you might contribute your own ideas…and collectively we might come up with some interesting thoughts. Ray, we have spoken at length about this topic and I know, having read your work and as a well-known futurist, you have firm ideas about evolution and how man will sustain himself in the future. I am particularly interested in your thoughts on nutrition.

Ray Kurzweil:…indeed. In my book, *"The Singularity Is Near: When Humans Transcend Biology"* I set forth…

Mao Tse Dong: Singula…..What?

Ray Kurzweil: Singularity. It is a conceptual, technological-evolutionary jump whereby we, as humans will be able to augment our bodies and minds with technology. I describe the singularity as resulting from a combination of three important technologies of the 21st century: genetics, nanotechnology, and robotics (including artificial intelligence) and merging them with our bodies. Once we have achieved such a state, we, I mean our new semi-biological selves, will control the aging process be smarter by a factor of trillions and more.

Mao: (aghast) You are a reactionary…and I will have the Red Guard cast you down without hope of rehabilitation! (looking around, alarmed) Where's Zhou Enlai…?

Bromme 柯博明 : Easy Mao, you can't…first you are dead, second, China is slightly different today.

Ray Kroc[56]: (curious, as he spears at the fish with his chopsticks) ok, ok…but what does this all have to do with food?

Bromme 柯博明: Good question….I was hoping you would ask… Ray?

Ray Kurzweil: Yes. My friend and colleague, Robert A. Freitas, has pioneered certain nanotechnologies and designed robotic replacements for human blood cells that perform hundreds of times more effectively than their biological counterparts. Freitas's respirocytes could enable an olympic sprinter to run for 15 minutes

---

56 Ray Kroc: (October 5, 1902 – January 14, 1984) was an American businessman. He joined McDonald's in 1954 and built it into the most successful fast food operation in the world.

without breathing. Some of his other inventions are nano-bots which are mechanical versions of propulsive cilia...the necessary nourishment could be delivered by similar micro-bots, each loaded with vitamins and other necessary nutrients, directly into cells.

Julia Child[57]: (horrified and shrill).....*Mon Dieu!*

Ray Kroc: (impatient and Texan-like)...Where's my answer, Kurzweil...?

Mao: (interrupting) I like you Ray...Ray Kroc....*Kampei!* (Mao raises his glass of Moutai[58] in a respectful toast to Ray Kroc)... you...(extending his long, indicting finger directly at Kurzweil... solemnly)...the other Ray, this one...I do not like....

Ray Kurzweil: (unconcerned)...Ok...there is already an innovative little micro-machine with micro-teeth embedded in a jaw that opens and closes to trap individual cells and then implant them with substances such a DNA, proteins or drugs. These same nano-machines could carry the precise nutrients, including all the phytochemicals necessary for the optimal health of any individual not just an elderly person. Eventually, we won't need to bother with extracting nutrients from food at all. Nutrients will be introduced directly in the bloodstream by special metabolic nano-bots and adjacent sensors, using Wi-Fi technology, will provide dynamic information on the nutrients we need from time to time.

---

57 Julia Child: August 15, 1912 – August 13, 2004) was an American chef, author, and television personality. She is recognized for bringing French cuisine to the American public with her debut cookbook, Mastering the Art of French Cooking, and her subsequent television programs, the most notable of which was The French Chef, which premiered in 1963.

58 Moutai is a high proof, clear spirit made of sorghum. It is expensive and popular among business elite and politicians in China. It is not, however, typically served in nursing homes.

Julia: (bereft and, yes, shrill)....Plus de nourriture? Plus de *boeuf bourguignon*?

Mao: Mei-you[59]...

Ray Kroc: (on a roll...gesturing with his hands in the air) I like it, Kurzweil. I see it now...."Happy nano-meals"...."nano-nutrients for the masses"....Hey, Mao..?

Mao: (attentive!) Yes, Comrade!

Ray Kroc: Let's cut a deal....How about licensing me to create happy nano-meals for your people?

Mao: (dismissive) ah...er...I'm not that good with economics.... better speak to Deng Xiao Peng.

Bromme 柯博明: Wait a minute, let's not get ahead of ourselves here......I am not sure I buy this whole thing about no more food.

Ray Kurzweil: Oh, no...You misunderstand....we still have food....it is just different and frankly better for you. At the same time the nano-bots nourish you, they destroy pathogens like bacteria, viruses and cancer cells.

Bromme 柯博明: Sure....but I love the smell of apple pie cooking in a busy kitchen!

Ray Kurzweil: Ok...your new non-biological self will stimulate your olfactory senses with whatever scent you most desire.

---

59 English translation of this Mandarin phrase means: no, none.

Julia: (appalled)...Quel horreur!

Bromme 柯博明: I am not sure I like that....the idea of being semi-human...I have grown accustomed to my limitations...and I like eating.

Ray Kurzweil: Ah...perhaps our differences lie in the way we value machines...

Aubrey de Grey[60]: (chewing a mouthful of healthy bok-choy) May I....

Bromme 柯博明: Please...Tell us what you have for us!

Aubrey: (chewing) Frankly...all this is inevitable. At some point in the near future, as a result of the technologies already in place and given the speed of further innovations, humans will begin to live longer. The first person to live to 300 is likely only 15 years older than the first person to live to 1000. I am not sure I agree with the extent to which Ray is suggesting we will become less biological, but exceedingly long life is very close...decades at most.

Mao: (gleeful) My Party will live forever...an everlasting dynasty!

Bromme 柯博明: Don't bet on it...Mao.

---

60 Aubrey de Grey: born 20 April 1963 is an English author and well known theoretician in the field of gerontology, and the Chief Science Officer of the SENS Foundation. He is editor-in-chief of the academic journal Rejuvenation Research, author of The Mitochondrial Free Radical Theory of Aging (1999) and co-author of Ending Aging (2007). De Grey is perhaps best known for his view that human beings could, in theory, live to lifespans far in excess of that which any authenticated cases have lived to today.

Mao: Well, at least my people could…well, we already have a population problem. If people could live forever then we wouldn't have to resort to other more radical policies being contemplated… we could reduce population growth…

Bromme 柯博明: (cutting Mao off)…and we know all too well about these.

Aubrey: All the core knowledge to develop engineered negligible senescence, or halting degeneration of the body and brain, is within our capabilities at presence. Once we have successfully applied these technologies to, say, a mouse, and achieve a "robustly rejuvenated mouse" or a mouse that is functionally younger than before treatment, we are no less than 10 years away from a human application.

Ray Kroc: (uninterested and dismissive) I want to get back to my Happy nano-meal…

Julia: (incensed) Happy meals?…An insult to the Culinary Arts and an abomination of health!

Bromme 柯博明: Naturally, Ray.

Ray Kurzweil: (apologetically) Mr. Kroc, I see what you are getting at…and as an inventor I appreciate your entrepreneurism… but, eating will no longer be the social experience we know it today and we certainly won't spend time driving too fast "nano-meal" locations. Nourishment will be delivered as downloadable attachments to messages which we will be able to receive directly.

Ray Kroc: (not quite understanding the email concept) uh...ok...but these attachments will be purchased somewhere and made somehow...that's where I come in...!

Ray Kurzweil: True...but all that we need for that part of us that remains biological will be ordered online and prepared by machines without human intervention. Money in the sense that you know it today will no longer exist.

Ray Kroc: (crestfallen but relentless) ....I know there MUST be a way...

Julia: (indignant and still shrill) You two, Ray Kurzweil and Aubrey de Grey, are quite a pair....This is a very frightening vision you offer! *Extraordinaire!*

Bromme 柯博明: Well, there are moral and ethical implications.... right guys?

Ray Kurzweil: (supremely confident) To be sure, but they should subside once the benefits are made apparent.

Aubrey:....Not to mention the overwhelming desire that many humans have to live much longer. This will negate any objections I can foresee.

Bromme 柯博明: According to you both, it sounds like my business, senior living...geriatrics....gerontology... not to mention the subject of this essay, "Geriatric Nutrition" has a limited future...?

Mao: (forlorn, sensing the end of my reverie) Xiao-jie![61]…Can I get some more Moutai?

Aubrey: (smiling at Mao) It's a dying industry….no pun intended. If people can live for centuries…there is no real need for nursing homes.

Ray Kurzweil: Or food for that matter….Indeed, it is an obsolete business.

Julia: (exasperated) Well, I have *never*…! I shall eat this meal and chew every morsel as if it were my last...I will starve before I download any meal into my body nor will I willingly consume any robot!

Dessert

I left my imaginary lunch not having eaten much; I was too concerned with what I had imagined. As I strolled down Fuxing Lu towards my apartment, I thought….inevitable?...nourishment via nano-bots?....thousands of micro-machines crawling about my gut feeding me? No more cool, juicy watermelon on a hot summer's day….no more crispy BBQ chicken wings on Superbowl Sunday? More importantly, no more Chef Chu…..and everything that comes with his food. After all, how do you lovingly inject someone with 50,000 food-packed micro-bots? Seriously, I can see some disgruntled former chef laid off from his job at a 5 star restaurant; made redundant by food carrying micro-bots and now unemployable. In a fit of rage he creates some malware which infects Kurzweil's micro-machines…they go berserk with horrific consequences; devouring their host from the inside. Semi-humans

---

61 Waitress!

of the future will joke and say the former chef went "buffet". But in all seriousness, motivation to eat may no longer an issue as all the nutrition we need would be absorbed...but I wonder if motivation to live will be the issue in this frightening brave new world of nutrition.

No doubt there are benefits to this scenario, especially the idea that dietetic deficiencies could be determined real time. And there are probably enormous cost savings to be had and the difficulties with delivery of food to those who would otherwise go malnourished could be alleviated if not eliminated. But all the rest of the Kurzweil/ de Grey future-world leaves me with a belly ache; perhaps there is

an alternative, middle of the road solution where we don't need to become less biological and the nano-bots are kept to a minimum. I certainly hope so.

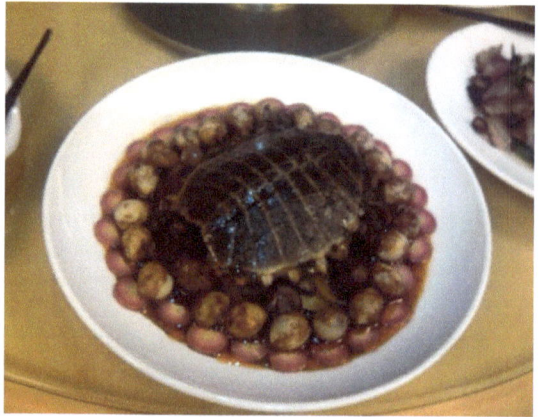

Figure 45 Braised Turtle

It seems to me that Chef Chu, had he not been the master chef at the Grand Hotel in Taipei, he would have made a marvelous and caring geriatric nutritionist. How do we emulate Chef Chu, with all his love and caring if we feed and are fed by robots? How do micro-machines nourish the soul? Being semi-human or at least being fed by cellular sized machines is not a transcendental concept, in fact I find it wholly uninspiring, cold and quite morbid. Nevertheless, beware: this may well be where food, ageing and the future intersect especially with our love of technology. Unrestrained population growth, technology improving at ever faster rates of growth, an unceasing fascination with longevity and chronic food shortages in many parts of the world may thrust this or some similar future upon us unknowingly; our ability to find solutions (to these challenges) which reinforce our humanity, not lessen it, will be evidence of our attempts to rise above our limits not as semi-biological entities but as humans in full.

Intermission: Livable Hong Kong
中场片段: 宜居香港

At the south-eastern tip of China, before you get to the island of Hainan, the mighty Pearl River forms a vast delta and empties her warm waters into the South China Sea. Tucked up inside this delta is a near perfectly protected, deep water harbor known as Victoria. Victoria's

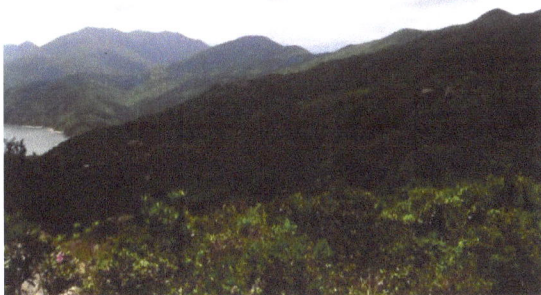

Figure 46 Dragon's Back hiking trail, Hong Kong

primary port of call is Hong Kong; one of over 262 islands in the greater Pearl River estuary. Hong Kong covers a total of area of over 1,100 square kilometers with less than 25% of its total area developed and a population of about 7 million; roughly the size of New York City.

Hong Kong is a Special Administrative Region of the People's Republic of China. When the British lease expired in 1997, China assumed sovereignty under a 'one country, two systems' principle. Hong Kong's effective ruling instrument is the Hong Kong SAR

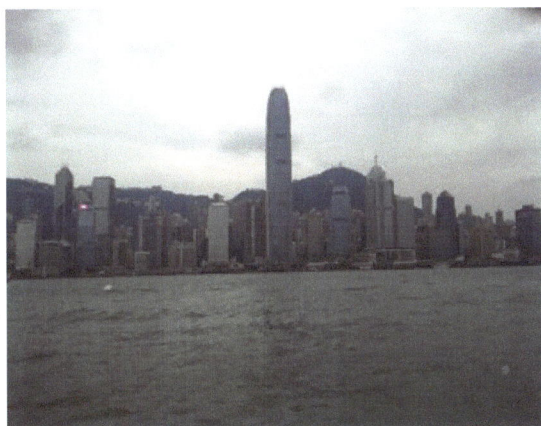

Figure 47 View of Central from the Star Ferry crossing Victoria Harbor

constitution; a document that ensures the current political situation, as the British left it, will remain in effect for 50 years.

Like a lot of big, highly urbanized international cities, Hong Kong is a city of contradictions; and a contradiction on every level imaginable – political: with the one country, two systems concept, social: the locals and the Westerners could not be more different, economic: the disparity between rich and poor is apparent on every street corner. But as contradictions go, Hong Kong's are not inconsistent or incongruous. It is just a jumble of opposing forces and competing powers which engage peacefully and coexist productively; just like they have done for nearly 200 years. These contradictions form a lovable cultural mosaic; a very agreeable montage of western and eastern influences set on a canvass long ago woven with British organization; Hong Kong has a vibe and a groove for everyone.

Another pleasant ambiguity is that 25 minutes away from Central, one can be in the midst of awe inspiring wilderness. For example, an afternoon hike along Dragon's Back trail is no further than a 20 minute subway trip to Chai Wan and then a 5 minute bus ride: all from downtown Hong Kong. It is a strenuous and refreshing hike, snakes, spiders abound, which clears one's lungs of Central's soot. Views from the top of the Shek-O peninsula are breath-taking: to the south and east one has wide, blue ocean panoramas and to the west and north you can gaze upon the towering green mountains of Hong Kong Island. It takes 3.5 hours to hike Dragon's Back; at the end of the trail, one can relax and drink a cool Lychee nut juice at Big Wave Bay and watch Chinese surfers ride the big blue rollers of the South China Sea.

I took this hike in late January and less than thirty minutes after my last step on the wild Shek-O peninsula, I was back in Central;

emerging from the subway and confronted once again with the cement jungle that is downtown Hong Kong. The cool breeze of the mountains was now replaced by the dank humidity of urban infrastructure. But, no need for further climbing, I think…I am in Soho…and I hop on the modern outdoor, elevated escalator at Queen's Road which easily transports me back up the steep trek to Mid-Levels. As I glide higher and higher, I watch the street scene pass below me noticing my hiking boots are crusted with a contrasting mix

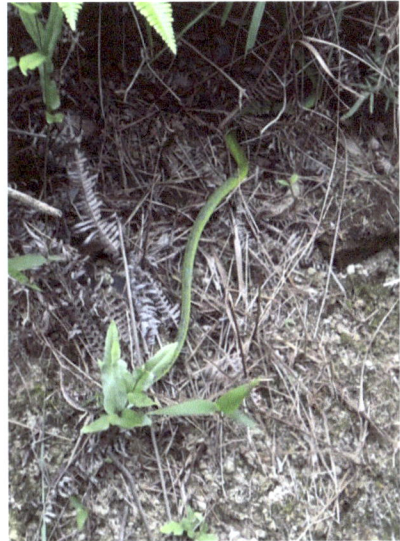

Figure 48 Venomous Bamboo snake along Dragon's Back trail, Shek-O

of Shek-O mountain mud and Big Wave Bay sand. My tired legs appreciate the convenience of the moving sidewalk. Once again back in the dizzy heights that surround Central, I marvel about my afternoon: urban escalators to wilderness trails and back again in about 4 hours. The proximity of them is precisely the type of contradiction that is characteristic of Hong Kong…it makes the city eminently habitable and charmingly unpredictable.

I hope there will never be an escalator on Dragon's Back; needless to say that would be a very unappealing contradiction.

The Delicious Tea of Shou Xing
寿星的中国养老预测

"There have never been a people more purely artist, and therefore more purely lover, than the Chinese...", General Yen in
The Bitter Tea of General Yen

General Yen's platitude, whether true or not, could be debated with convincing argument pro and con ad infinitum. Yet, it should be without doubt that 5,000 years of Chinese culture have produced a legacy of beautiful art. Art breeds compassion and the care of the elderly is brewed with compassionate, sympathetic kindnesses and steeped in technological specialties. Despite the chaotic situation senior living finds itself in China, the Chinese have the fundamental skills especially the patience, in abundance, to create a geriatric care culture over time with little intervention from the West.

The Bitter Tea of General Yen is the most unusual talkie effort of director Frank Capra. Barbara Stanwyck stars as Megan Davis, the fiancée of an American missionary who is sent to spread the good word in China. During a military uprising, Stanwyck and her fiancé inadvertently wander into forbidden territory while helping a group of orphans escape. The couple is forcibly detained by refined warlord General Yen (played by Swedish actor Nils Asther), who relies upon the financial advice of wayward American expatriate Jones (played by Walter Connolly). Yen is overcome with desire at the sight of the beautiful Davis; who is at first repulsed by his attentions but later finds herself strangely drawn in by his charisma. During the film, General Yen's fortunes wane and everyone but Jones and Davis desert him; he for no other reason than greed and she due to an increased attraction to the General. Yen's army lieutenants betray him leading to the loss of his treasure, his army disbands, and with no further options and suffering under the belief he has lost Davis as well, he drinks a poison tea. This film is all about the tensions between Western idealism and Chinese pragmatism.

This was the first film to play at the newly constructed Radio City Music Hall and it was scheduled for a

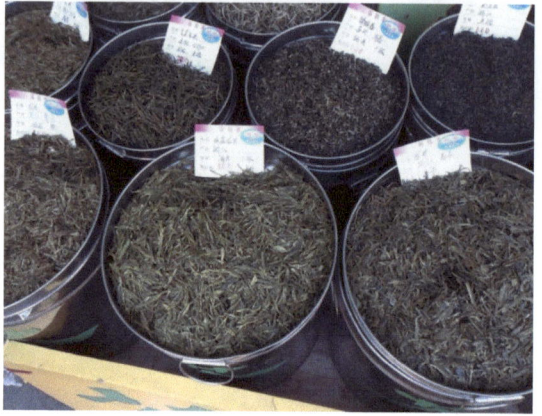

Figure 49 Barrels of tea in a market in Shanghai

minimum two-week run, but the theater cancelled it after eight days resulting in a certain loss; few people came to view the film despite good to fair critical reviews. More interestingly, the film was banned in parts of the British Empire for miscegenation. When Columbia Pictures sought to reissue the film in 1950, the Production Code Administration[62] was adamant that the film's characterizations of Americans and Chinese, specifically the scene in which the heroine offers herself to a Chinese man, were "very questionable"; Columbia caved and the film was not re-released. Capra and Stanwyck were both dismayed by the racist reaction and argued the artistic merits of the film, claiming the depiction was simply a natural outcome of passions molded by tumultuous times. To no avail, the film was confined to a basement vault of failed Hollywood films and has since been long forgotten.

---

62 Hollywood's self-censoring body formed in 1934.

A special brew

The practice of preparing and drinking of tea in some parts of China[63] has risen to a highly refined art form, called not surprisingly the Gong-Fu method of tea preparation. It is steeped in ceremony and ritual with no fewer than 8 and sometimes 12 distinct practices from the selection of the tea to warming of the cup and eventually sipping the tea and, of course, offering gracious compliments to the host for a sublime experience. Each aspect of the ritual has been named, in distinctly Chinese style, with exceedingly poetic phrases: Tea Masters call the placing of tea into the pot "the black dragon enters the palace"; rinsing the teapot prior and pouring hot water onto the tea is known as "bathing the immortal twice"; and when the drinking cup is carefully balanced over a special scent cup, specialists in the art of tea refer to this as "the dragon and phoenix in auspicious union"...this is China after all.

On a chilly November afternoon last fall the weather in Shanghai was threatening an early winter. I was walking from a client's office after a meeting regretting not having a warmer coat and as I strolled down Huangpi Lu not far from People's Square the afternoon chill got to me. I decided to stop by a tea house well known for tasseography[64] and warm up with a cup of soothing Longjing cha. I pushed the heavy wood door open, it swiveled and squeaked on wood pegs set into a granite hearth; this was unusually old construction for this part of Shanghai, I thought. As I entered the shop, I was further surprised to notice that it was very small for a tea house; five tables set out in a pentagon shape each with two stools, in the center of the room was a cast iron heater; its fire warmed the room nicely. I moved past the heater and sat at the furthest table, set my bag down and waited for someone to come.

---

63 Some report that the art of tea drinking is most traditional in Taiwan as during the Cultural Revolution much of the art of Gong-fu tea described here was banned.

64 The art of telling the future with tea leaves.

It was a sturdy table despite its age; the top was full of deep scars now filled with old wax from ages of polishing, one could tell it had a long history. I looked around the room: placed on the table to my left was a bowl brimming with fresh peaches, and set on the table to my right was a pumpkin gourd lying on its side; leaning against the front wall just to the right of the door was a long staff with a curious carving on top. Two windows on the front wall were framed with old wooden casements and the glass was nearly covered with beads of condensation preventing a clear view in or out.

Not a minute later a smiling old man with a long smooth white beard appeared from behind a curtain which hid a side room. He wore a flowing orange silk gown imprinted with stylized Chinese characters for long life. The sleeves were long and wide and they fully concealed his hands. He shuffled across the room and over to my table. He looked like an old Mandarin mystic; he was vaguely familiar to me.

He spoke in a simple way with a heavy accent. Bowing slightly he greeted me with a wide smile,

"Pleased to welcome 柯 博 明 to humble tea house. Recommend daily special tea for enjoyment on cold afternoon?"

I nodded and thanked him. "Ah, sure, that would be fine."

The old man shuffled back behind the curtain and reappeared almost instantly carrying an old pot, a cup and small bowl. His cloth slippers made a swoosh-swoosh sound on the brick floor as scurried back across the room, the orange robe he wore swaying as he moved. He placed the teapot, cup and bowl on the table and in the same motion, he sat down on the stool across from me.

As he was adjusting his posture, I interrupted the moment, "I don't need my fortune read…just the tea, thank you."

The old man smiled and persisted, "Ah, young man must understand direction of future, important for business and for life." Not looking at me, he began to arrange the cup, bowl and teapot.

I responded, "Thank you…really, but it isn't what I want."

"Patience, 柯博明, patience…is most important ingredient for good tea and good future…let black dragon wake up", the old man pointed at the teapot and imparted some Gong-Fu terminology meaning that the tea was steeping.

We sat there for five minutes. The old man remained perfectly still, staring straight ahead…smiling…and then, suddenly, like some battery-powered toy whose on-switch had just been flipped, he poured out a cup of tea. Dozens of leaves spilled out of the spout and into my cup as the steam rose and curled around in the space between us. The warmth of the room was comforting and I began to relax despite the old man's persistence.

"Learn about future of business…much has been discussed…but no one understands direction. Drink and enjoy tea now…pour leaves into bowl",… the old man was solemn but his smile never left his face.

I was growing dismayed with his insistence, "Please, I just want to drink my tea, ok?"

I took a long sip of Longjing and, looking at this oddity of an old man, I began to protest again as I placed my cup back down on the table. But my aim was off and I hit the teapot instead; the tea spilled out of my cup and the tea leaves scattered onto the bowl he had placed in front of me.

"Darn"...I mumbled.

"No!..how auspicious!", the old man exclaimed. "Take look at tea leaves...see arrangement of future business".

The old man's hands appeared from under the folds of his sleeves and he rolled them together at chest height as he studied the leaves, his eyes darting back and forth among the Rorschach-like pattern left in the bowl. He mumbled to himself for a moment then looked up at me.

"Ah, 柯博明, I see complicated future for China senior living business...care of China old persons will be good but path is hard... but you can see clearly..." he spoke as he studied the leaves more.

"Explain", I said, now curious as to his thoughts.

The old man looked up at me with his permanent grin. Here is a transcription of his 9 predictions for the senior care industry in China:

1) *Western operator involvement* – Real, meaning economically feasible, opportunities for Western operators will be few and far in between. Those that manage successful ventures will have invested significantly in China and fully localized their operation which means significant upfront expenditures...and these operators will be just as vulnerable to the human resource poaching as the local operators. Acceptance of a China CCRC and the life style living concept is 15 years in the future.

2) *Branding* – Branding will aid Westerners in their effort to win business but ultimately, one's guanxi will be what makes a venture successful in China. If you don't know what this is or its development isn't a priority on your agenda, go home... seriously.

3) *Transactions* - All ventures will be/must be structured with equal economics between partners or they will not work.

4) *Deal duration* - Expect at least 5-7 year horizon to positive cash flow and more likely 7-10 years. Total transaction life will be 10-15 years.

5) *Severe human resource poaching* – Make no mistake; once you train your staff you will lose them to a local competitor who pays them just a nickel more. The absolute lack of a local pool of human resources is and will continue to retard meaningful growth in the industry. But bear in mind that the problem isn't just the lack of skilled or competent workers; the problem is compounded by the simple fact that health care jobs, such as nurses or health care workers, are a low status occupation that offer no pride in one's work.

6) *Continued industry segmentation* – Aged care or skilled nursing for all economic cohorts will thrive. Attempts at independent living development will continue to be troubled especially the campus style projects, unless developers undertake significant market research in advance of construction and formulate design based on conjoint analysis; something that Chinese builders are reluctant to do. Home care will grow but will be constrained by dearth of human resources.

7) *Harmful regulations and legislation* - The CPC and provincial authorities will react to negative events, all of which inevitably occur, with overly protective legislation

that sets the industry back and hinders progress. These events are very likely given the unregulated circumstances under which builders create senior care projects at present. These negative events might be as follows:

    a. Failure of a developer to manage his financial accounts properly and is therefore unable to refund residents their deposits at the end of their lease.

    b. A life-safety issue, be it a fire, building collapse or other.

    c. Uncovering of widespread abuse/neglect of elderly.

8) *Health care information technology* – The emerging HiT industry will offer significant economies for the rapidly developing Chinese health care system and enable broad geriatric care coverage for the elderly, wealthy, middle income and poor alike, via remote monitoring of vital systems. With HiT both the quality of care and availability will rise for elderly and it will be complimentary to either facility living or the home care alternative.

And finally:

9) *A new concept in senior care for China* – There will emerge, in the next three years, a concept for elderly care incorporating both modern senior services and aspects of Chinese culture that have endured for centuries. The concept will be immediately acceptable to the elderly and offer their children a cost effective way to manage their parents. This concept has come out of my nearly 4 years in this business here in China, watching various models come and go, seeing how the western style CCRC's have failed here and concluding that the best model is to provide the Chinese with something that fits within the perimeter of their cultural expectations. I am not disclosing this model, but if you want to learn more, contact me.

Then after speaking for what must have been 45 minutes, the old man simply sat back on his stool. I thanked him and attempted to pay my bill; he adamantly refused. As I stood he stood and we walked across the room together. I opened the door noticing that the squeak of wooden hinge on granite was now strangely gone. As I left the tea house the old man bowed; I nodded but was distracted…I stepped out and found myself lost in deep thought about both the wisdom of patience and his predictions of the future.

The wind had picked up along Huangpi Lu and a light drizzle was now falling making the slate sidewalk slick. Headlights from approaching cars reflected off the wet streets and made the asphalt glow. I gingerly crossed the road and looked back at the tea house. The condensation had lifted off the windows and I could see the old man standing behind the window on the left, now holding the staff with that self-amused, worriless grin looking right at me; I now recognized him and knew who he was. For the first time in the 4 years that I had been working in China I felt I had a clear understanding of what the industry needed and where it was going. Feeling satisfied and appreciative towards my good friend Shou for all he had revealed, I buttoned my coat,

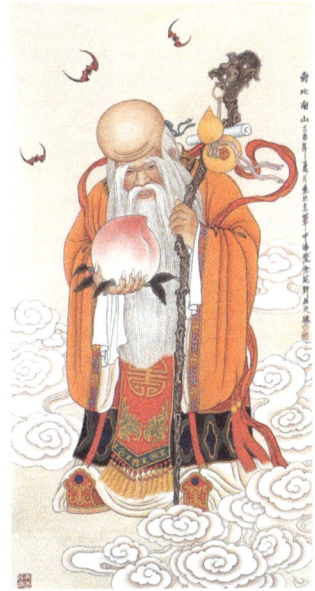

Figure 50 Shou Xing - Deity of Longevity

crossed Nanjing Xi Lu, walked into People's Square and back homeward.

Let it steep

Megan Davis learned an important lesson in her drama with General Yen and one that is a universal truth which can be applied to much, if not all, of what we as Westerners must accept about the Chinese if we are to work, successfully, in China. Ultimately, she was unable to change General Yen and her specific case, Western moral standards and ideals of Christian forgiveness were wasted on Yen's deeply ingrained Confucian ideology and innate practicality. In order for her to get along and survive, she needed to adhere to and accept his ways of doing things. Similarly, Western geriatricians and senior living experts must understand that Western ways of practicing the art of Gerontology may be absorbed by the Chinese but they will alter these concepts to suit their own tastes and culture. No matter how much one tries to impose a methodology on the Chinese, if it is not congruent with their own sense of what is culturally appropriate for them, it will be discarded irrespective of how crucial any one particular lesson or technique may be to the field of Geriatrics. The Chinese will always choose the least complicated, most economical solution for any particular challenge and then fill it with sufficient ambiguity so that it is only comprehended by them. This may seem simplistic and obvious, but I assure you it has deep and consequential meaning for every aspect of business life in China and its application is without exception.

The last twelve essays along with the intermissions have covered a lot of ground. From China's elder demographics, to health care technology opportunities, a little behavioral science, some human resources, a market study, nutritional information and with this final chapter, a look into the future at the pleasure of Shou Xing. In retrospect, I believe the collective information imparted in all essays convey a realistic picture of not just where this industry is at present but how it gets to where it is going and, most importantly, what it will be like when it has arrived. Just remember, the best way to do business in China is like the best way to drink tea...be patient and enjoy it, you cannot hurry; and if you rush, it will be a bitter experience.

Thank you.

About the Author

Bromme Hampton Cole 柯 博 明 was born in New Orleans, USA but having lived on the island of Manhattan for many years, he is much more a peripatetic New Yorker than a son of the Big Easy. He has also lived a good portion of his life abroad in such countries as France, Taiwan, Colombia and now lives in China; he is fluent in French, Spanish and Mandarin. An incurable adventurer, he is a Mason and part of the proud Dutch diaspora. Professionally, he has been involved in the business of health care for most of his career, from banking to investment and now from as a consultant and advisor to similarly minded Asian businessmen. He is equally passionate about his client's success as he is in providing a decent future for the elderly in an ageing world. When he isn't in Asia managing his health care businesses, he can be found in New York City: recharging in the East Room with the gentlemen of 69th street, at Collation on 23rd street or reveling in the simple joy of flying kites with his family on Asparagus Beach in Amagansett, NY.

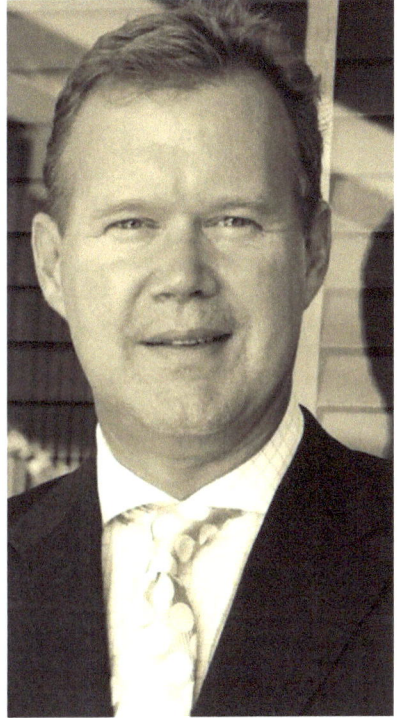

This is his first published book.

`关于作者

柯博明（Bromme Hampton Cole）出生于美国新奥尔良，在曼哈顿岛生活了很多年。所以他更像是巡游的纽约客，而不是新奥尔良式的大快活家。他还在法国，哥伦比亚，台湾和中国生活过相当长的时间，会说流利的法语，西班牙语和中文。作为一个执着的探索者，他笃信人类平等，这是源自他1632年移居曼哈顿的荷兰祖先的根本原则。从专业上柯先生多年一直专注于医疗领域，包括相关的金融，投资业务，还有现在为亚洲商务领袖提供的顾问咨询服务。他对于帮助客户取得成功以及促进长者服务的发展都赋予着同样的热忱。当柯总不在亚洲管理医疗业务的时候，他通常会在纽约六十九街东厅与绅士友人交流，或在二十三街与兄弟们相聚，或与家人在纽约阿默甘西特的芦笋海滩尽享放风筝的简单快乐。

这是他出版的第一本书。

Enter the Ageing Dragon...
中国龙进入高龄化社会…

With a Preface by Mark Spitalnik, CEO - China Senior Care

Today, China's elderly population is approaching a staggering 170 million and in 2025 it will exceed 250 million. This demographic fact coupled with a growing Chinese middle class, have combined to make the senior living business one of the most dynamic new industries on the Mainland. There is a lot that Westerners can do here…and a lot they will not be able to do. The extent to which Western experts in geriatrics and those in the business of health care can participate in this extraordinary industry depends on one's ability to do business the Chinese-way. And what doing business the Chinese-way actually means is not easily defined but requires a cultural awareness that comes only with time spent in China and, of course, that elusive quality of effective cross-cultural relationships, patience. _Enter the Ageing Dragon…_ is an insightful chronicle of one man's experience in the senior living business in China from its very inception…his views on its future development and more importantly, how he was successful. A gifted story teller with intuitive multicultural business instincts, the author artfully narrates the story through the entertaining lens of classical movies about China.

Advance praise from global senior living industry leaders!

"…Cole's informed and often humorous observations on senior living in China are both timely and extremely helpful…he helps us understand this unique market!"
BRAD PERKINS FAIA MRAIC AICP— CHAIRMAN/CEO - PERKINS EASTMAN (USA)

柯博明对中国老年人困境的深刻理解，把握和同情让我深受感动。这种困境是任何人都不应漠视的
"I was deeply moved by Bromme's understanding, profound grasp and broad sympathy toward the plight of aged population in China"
YUE TANG唐越 — PARTNER, JUNEHE LAW FIRM君合律师事务所（CHINA）

"Félicitations Bromme!…une brillante analyse!"
PASCAL BRUNELET — CEO, COLISÉE PATRIMOINE (FRANCE)

"An immensely valuable resource for senior living in China…very insightful…prescient…Bromme understands China to a T!"
KEVIN RYAN — CEO, WATERBROOK SENIOR LIVING (AUSTRALIA)

"…I found Cole's new book not only entertaining but also quite informative!
DAVID FRESHWATER — CHAIRMAN, THE FRESHWATER GROUP (USA)

为长者服务！
Patient Lao Wai Publications
China Senior Living and Hampton Hoerter China